Christopher Gill

HEROIC MEASURES

STUDIES IN
ANCIENT MEDICINE

EDITED BY

JOHN SCARBOROUGH

PHILIP J. VAN DER EIJK
ANN HANSON
NANCY SIRAISI

VOLUME 30

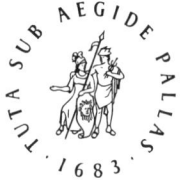

HEROIC MEASURES

Hippocratic Medicine in the Making of Euripidean Tragedy

BY

JENNIFER CLARKE KOSAK

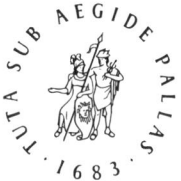

BRILL
LEIDEN · BOSTON
2004

Cover Illustration: Telephus holding the baby Orestes. The Nazzano Painter, *Calyx-krater*. Italic, Latin, Faliscan, Late Classical Period, about 380-360 B.C. Photograph © 2004 Museum of Fine Arts, Boston.

This book is printed on acid-free paper.

Library of Congress Cataloging-in-Publication Data

Kosak, Jennifer Clarke.
   Heroic measures : Hippocratic medicine in the making of Euripidean tragedy / by Jennifer Clarke Kosak.
      p. cm. — (Studies in ancient medicine, ISSN 0925-1421 ; v. 30)
      Includes bibliographical references (p.) and index.
      ISBN 90-04-13993-1 (acid-free paper)
      1. Euripides—Knowledge—Medicine. 2. Literature and medicine—Greece—History—To 500. 3. Medicine, Greek and Roman. 4. Hippocrates—Influence. 5. Medicine in literature. 6. Tragedy. I. Title. II. Series.

PA3978.K57 2004
882'.01—dc22
                                                                                        2004054524

ISSN   0925–1421
ISBN   90 04 13993 1

PRINTED IN THE NETHERLANDS

CONTENTS

ACKNOWLEDGEMENTS

This study is a revised version of the dissertation I completed in 1994 at the University of Michigan in Ann Arbor. I am grateful to the Department of Classical Studies and the Horace H. Rackham School of Graduate Studies for financial support throughout my time there. I also express my deep appreciation to the members of my doctoral committee, Ann Ellis Hanson, Ludwig Koenen, James I. Porter, Arlene Saxonhouse, and Ruth Scodel (who served as my advisor) for their help during the writing of the dissertation and for their suggested improvements. I hope I have been able to incorporate some of their fine ideas into the book in its current form. I owe special thanks to Ruth Scodel, who was my first Greek instructor when I was an undergraduate, and who, with her encyclopedic knowledge of Greek literature and her ability to see quickly the heart of an argument, has been a ready source of suggestions and an invaluable sounding board for my ideas over the years. I also owe a particular debt of gratitude to Ann Hanson, who not only introduced me to the riches of the Hippocratic Corpus but also, with her typical generosity, read a recent version of the present work with meticulous care, correcting errors and making many helpful remarks (any errors that remain are, of course, my responsibility); her help and guidance have been invaluable. In addition, I would like to thank the members of the departments of Classics at Emory University, Rutgers University, and, above all, Barbara Weiden Boyd, Jim Higginbotham and Irene Polinskaya, my colleagues at Bowdoin College, who have provided support and encouragement over the course of my itinerant career. At various times, Elizabeth Craik and Heinrich von Staden have heard and reacted to some of my ideas with careful suggestions, and I thank each of them for their interest. I am grateful to Michiel Klein Swormink at Brill for his patient assistance. Finally, I give thanks to my parents, sisters, husband and children for their commitment to the arts and humanities and for their belief in the value of books.

ABBREVIATIONS

In the text, I have used the most common English titles for ancient works. In the notes, I have generally used full titles or the abbreviations found in standard English reference works (e.g., *Oxford Classical Dictionary*; *LSJ*).

Abbreviated titles for the works of the Hippocratic Corpus:

Aer.	*Airs, Waters, Places*
Affect.	*Affections*
Aph.	*Aphorisms*
Ars	*The Art*
Artic.	*Articulations (also known as Joints)*
Coac.	*Coan Prenotions*
Decent.	*Decorum*
Dieb. Jud.	*Critical Days*
Epid. 1–7	*Epidemics 1–7*
Flat.	*Breaths*
Fract.	*Fractures*
Humor.	*Humors*
Intern.	*Internal Affections*
Jusj.	*The Oath*
Loc. Hom.	*Places in Man*
Morb. 1–4	*Diseases 1–4*
Morb. Sacr.	*On the Sacred Disease*
Morb. Mul 1–2	*Diseases of Women 1–2*
Nat. Hom.	*The Nature of Man*
Nat. Mul.	*The Nature of Women*
Nat. Puer.	*The Nature of the Child*
Prog.	*Prognostic*
Pror. 1–2	*Prorrhetics 1–2*
Reg. Acut.	*Regimen in Acute Diseases*
Steril.	*Barren Women*
Superf.	*Superfetation*

Ulc.	*Ulcers*
Vet. Med.	*On Ancient Medicine*
Reg. 1–3	*Regimen 1–3*

Abbreviated titles for works of Euripides and other tragedies frequently discussed:

Ag.	*Agamemnon*
PV	*Prometheus Bound*
Ant.	*Antigone*
OT	*Oedipus Tyrannus*
Phil.	*Philoctetes*
Cyc.	*Cyclopes*
Alc.	*Alcestis*
Med.	*Medea*
Heraclid.	*Heraclidae*
Hipp.	*Hippolytus*
Andr.	*Andromache*
Hec.	*Hecabe*
Supp.	*Suppliant Women*
El.	*Electra*
Her.	*Heracles*
IT	*Iphigeneia among the Taurians*
Hel.	*Helen*
Phoen.	*Phoenissae*
Or.	*Orestes*
Bac.	*Bacchae*
IA	*Iphigenia at Aulis*

Other abbreviations:

DK   H. Diels and W. Kranz, eds. *Die Fragmente der Vorsokratiker*. 6th edn. Berlin 1952.

LSJ   H.G. Liddell, R. Scott and H.S. Jones, *A Greek-English Lexicon*. 9th edition with Supplement. Oxford 1968.

TLG   *Thesaurus Linguae Graecae: a digital library of Greek literature*. Irving, CA 1996–.

TRAGEDY, MEDICINE AND SUFFERING
IN THE FIFTH CENTURY B.C.

Greek tragedy and Greek medical literature both treat forms of human suffering. They consider causes, seen and unseen, diagnoses, and cures. Greek tragedy and Greek medicine present to us 'ways of worldmaking'[1] in which we can see the patterns of thought and action that the Greeks—or at least some Greeks—felt explained their world and through which they tried to cope with the dangers and challenges confronting their existence. The conflicting claims of traditional or religious explanations of suffering and the newer philosophical or rationalist explanations can be discerned in fifth-century tragic and medical texts. The Greek dichotomy of *sôma* and *psychê*, body and soul, although to be sure rarely absolute, is reflected in the different emphases that the tragic and medical literatures place on physical and mental pain. Tragedy tends to focus on the suffering of the mind[2]—its characters feel the pain of grief, loss, death, and hardship—whereas medicine seeks for the most part to understand and ameliorate physical suffering, the suffering of the *sôma* as opposed to the *psychê*. The stylized metaphorical language of tragedy avoids mentioning the mundane diseases from which members of its audience surely suffered, whereas the prose works of the medical writers express little interest in myth or political interaction, locating the causes and cures of disease in the abiding laws of nature (*physis*). Yet fifth-century tragedy and Hippocratic medicine do intersect in several fundamental ways. If the Hippocratic doctor sees both external, physical forces (e.g., air, water, geography) and internal forces (e.g., blood, bile, water, phlegm) as essential elements in caus-

---

[1] This is the title of Nelson Goodman's book, *Ways of Worldmaking* (Indianapolis 1978), which analyzes the ways in which societies develop a conception of the world around them and its functions.

[2] Tragedy *does* focus on the body, to be sure, but the pain suffered by the body is often used as a visual representation of mental anguish or as a way in to discussion of a character's social relationships: for example, Sophocles' *Trachiniae* and *Philoctetes* graphically depict bodily suffering, yet at the same time, these plays focus not so much on healing the suffering of the body as on ways to relieve the suffering of the mind.

ing disease, tragedy too considers the relative weight of external (e.g., divine, social) and internal (e.g., hereditary, individual) factors in stories it represents. If medical writers consider interviews with patients, observation of symptoms, naming and classification of diseases, and prognoses as the most significant aspects of the doctor-patient relationship, so, too, do tragic figures discuss, probe, observe, diagnose, and predict the outcome of their particular situations (often—again like fifth-century doctors—with little success). If medical writers argue about methods of curing, such as harsh remedies like cutting and burning versus the softer approach of dietary regimen, or the virtues of allopathic medicine as opposed to homeopathic, so, too, do tragic characters consider resistance or capitulation, violence or reconciliation, removal or reintegration, as options that might resolve their situations. Significantly, tragedy often characterizes the difficulties it portrays as diseases and it seeks quite literally doctors (*iatroi*) and cures (*akea*).

The medical writers construct a portrait of the human body and its struggle with disease which can give us insight into the Greek sense of self at the end of the fifth century. If Greek temples, with their enduring strength, suggest to us a stable and unchanging landscape, if Greek religious rituals, carried out with faithful repetition year after year, suggest stable social institutions, history, drama, philosophy and medicine give us a view of the danger and unpredictability of the Greek world. The laws of nature may be fixed and eternal, but, according to philosophers such as Heraclitus, Empedocles, Anaxagoras and Democritus, they govern a world in motion, in which objects are not exactly as they appear, but rather phenomena arising from hidden, often conflicting forces. The medical texts show us the microcosm of the body, which many of the Hippocratic writers argue is in a precarious state of balance, its internal fluxes and organs subject to disruption by food and air, and sometimes even by the excess of one substance within the individual body from birth. The doctors' interest in discovering the primary causes of disease, their emphasis on categorization of diseases according to different symptoms, their belief in the importance of prediction (*prognôsis*), and their arguments over harsh and gentle methods of treatment correspond to similar preoccupations in other areas of contemporary culture. Yet the doctors' understanding of the workings of the human body was heavily based on theoretical principles, and they could often do very little when confronted by actual patients. Traditional medicine clearly played a powerful role in rationalist medical prescriptions. The pharmacological recipes suggested as cures surely had a long history in traditional Greek healing; the task of the Hippocratic doctor was to describe and categorize the different purposes of these drugs and to justify their use by argument and by appeal to theory. The influence of religious ideas, particularly the concept of pollution, can also be discerned in Hippocratic thinking, and indeed the healing cult of the god Asclepius provided a significant alternative to the care offered by the rationalist doctors. Hippocratic writers, with their use of terms and concepts such as *katharsis* (cleansing), *apostasis* (separation and/or expulsion) and *pharmakon* (drug), draw inspiration from traditional religious ideas. Thus, despite their insistence on non-divine, natural causality and rational principles of remedy, the fifth-century medical writers cannot escape certain ways of thinking about disease deeply embedded in Greek culture.

Greek tragedy, as an integral component of a major annual civic event, draws from and reflects upon the cultural mores and social concerns of the moment. By the end of the fifth century, the impact of the work of both the Presocratics and the sophists can be discerned in the plays produced by Sophocles and Euripides. Likewise, the overlapping and conflicting claims of rational and religious accounts of disease and suffering are reflected in the works of the tragic playwrights. These poets portray individuals suffering physically from various illnesses, which they and their companions seek to explain from both rationalistic and religious points of view. Divine causality competes with personal responsibility and natural causality in the case of the Euripidean Phaedra, Electra and Orestes, and the Sophoclean Heracles and Philoctetes, for example. Moreover, disease infects not only tragic individuals, but expands to epidemic proportions in tragic cities: thus, Thebes suffers from the plague in *Oedipus Tyrannus*, is 'sick with stasis' in *Heracles* (cf. 34, 272–273, 542–543), and demands the sacrifice of Menoeceus as a 'rescuing drug' (*pharmakon sôterias*, 893) in *Phoenissae*. Disease becomes a flexible metaphor in tragedy, suggestive of the breakdown of political unity, the corruption of leaders, and the rule of passion over reason. If medical voices argue that disease is increasingly subject to human understanding and thus to human control, tragic voices remain unconvinced by these rationalist claims even as they consider them.

Other ancient sources point to a second type of interaction between tragedy and medicine. After all, in his famous and controversial definition of tragedy in the *Poetics* (1449b24–28), Aristotle invokes a word significant in medicine—and in religion: the word *katharsis*. Aristotle argues that tragedy acts as a cathartic, in some way cleaning/purifying/

purging/relieving its spectators.[3] When Stoic philosophers took up the
question of tragedy's benefits and detriments, they, too, used medical models to explain the potentially positive aspects of tragedy in a
society. Martha Nussbaum has discussed how Epictetus, Chrysippus
and Plutarch apply medical analogies when prescribing the function
of tragedy appropriate for students of Stoic philosophy (and indeed,
for society in general). According to Stoic theory, the spectator who has
been properly trained to appreciate poetry 'doesn't suffer with the characters, he discerns their diseases and wants to heal them.'[4] In contrast
to Aristotelian theory, which relies upon identification between audience member and tragic character to achieve its effects, 'the spectator
now views himself as a kind of doctor-in-training of the soul.'[5] The idea
that tragedy is a form of medicine is found even in non-philosophical
contexts: a fragment from the comic poet Philippides seems to prescribe
Euripidean tragedy as an analgesic:

> ὅταν ἀτυχεῖν σοι συμπέσῃ τι, δέσποτα,
> Εὐριπίδου μνήσθητι, καὶ ῥᾴων ἔσῃ·
> οὐκ ἔστιν ὅστις πάντ' ἀνὴρ εὐδαιμονεῖ.
> εἶναι δ' ὑπόλαβε καὶ σε τῶν πολλῶν ἕνα.   (fr. 171 Kassel-Austin)

> Whenever it befalls you to be unlucky in some way, master,
> remember Euripides, and you'll feel better:
> there is no man who is fortunate in all ways,
> and understand that you are one of many.

---

[3] A tremendous analytical literature has grown up around this statement. Elizabeth
Belfiore (1992) has sought to interpret Aristotelian tragic *katharsis* in light of his usage
of the term in biological and medical contexts. Arguing against the common interpretation of Aristotelian tragic *katharsis* as a homeopathic process (the purging of pity and
fear by means of pity and fear), she suggests that *katharsis* consists rather in a purging
of harmful forms of emotion by means of an allopathic process; for Aristotle, tragedy
acts as an allopathic medicine which cleanses its spectators' minds and souls, purging
them of improper emotions and restoring the proper *krasis* of psychological health. She
writes: '... the phrase τῶν τοιούτων παθημάτων, 'such emotions,' in Aristotle's definition
of tragedy refers to emotions that are the same as pity and fear, and like them in kind,
but opposite in form. In tragic katharsis, the pre-existing emotional extreme of fear-
lessness and shamelessness is treated allopathically with the opposing extreme of tragic
emotion: *ekplexis*. The pity and fear aroused by tragedy effect a removal (katharsis) of
the opposite emotions 'concerning (tragic) pity and fear': fearless, shameless, aggressive,
thumetic emotions.' (p. 356) She continues, 'Like wine in Plato's *Laws*, tragedy, another
gift of Dionysos, is for Aristotle a drug to produce and renew *aidos* in the soul' (358).
In this form, tragic drama is useful for society, driving out inappropriate passions and
ennobling the members of the community.
[4] Nussbaum (1993) 141.
[5] Nussbaum (1993) 141.

If tragedy is a form of medicine, medical writers occasionally describe the hardships of the doctor's task in terms which seem to involve the doctor in the spectacle of a tragedy: the writer of *Breaths*, for example, begins his treatise thus:

εἰσί τινες τῶν τεχνέων αἳ τοῖσι μὲν κεκτημένοισίν εἰσιν ἐπίπονοι, τοῖσι δὲ χρεωμένοισιν ὀνήϊστοι, καὶ τοῖσι μὲν δημότῃσιν ξυνὸν ἀγαθόν, τοῖσι δὲ μεταχειριζομένοισί σφας λυπηραί. τῶν δὲ δὴ τοιούτων ἐστὶν τεχνέων καὶ ἣν οἱ Ἕλληνες καλέουσιν ἰητρικήν· ὁ μὲν γὰρ ἰητρὸς ὁρεῖ τὰ δεινά, θιγγάνει τὰ ἀηδέων, ἐπ᾽ ἀλλοτρίῃσί τε ξυμφορῇσιν ἰδίας καρποῦται λύπας· οἱ δὲ νοσέοντες ἀποτρέπονται διὰ τὴν τέχνην τῶν μεγίστων κακῶν, νούσων, λύπης, πόνων, θανάτου· πᾶσι γὰρ τουτέοισιν ἄντικρυς ἡ ἰητρική.

(1.1–3 Jouanna)

There are certain *technai* which are grievous for those who practice them, but beneficial for those who use them, and while they are a common good for the public, they are painful for those who actually do the handiwork. Belonging to such a group of *technai* is what the Greeks call the medical *technê*: for while the doctor sees terrible things and touches unpleasant ones and reaps his own personal and private pain in the sufferings of others, the sick are relieved by means of the *technê* from the greatest evils, diseases, grief, toils, death. Opposed to all these things is medical *technê*.

The doctor here acts both as a spectator, seeing terrible things (ὁρεῖ τὰ δεινά), and as a participant in the sufferings (ξυμφορῇσιν) of his patients. The author claims moreover that the skill of the doctor cures great evils which he defines as 'diseases, grief, toils, death,' evils very common in tragedy. Suffering from the suffering of others is a common topos in the fifth century. Thus, Gorgias echoes the sentiment of *Breaths*' author in his description of private pain suffered because of the pain of others: … ἐπ᾽ ἀλλοτρίων τε πραγμάτων καὶ σωμάτων εὐτυχίαις καὶ δυσπραγίας ἴδιόν τι πάθημα διὰ τῶν λόγων ἔπαθεν ἡ ψυχή (DK 82 B11 [9]: 'In the good fortune and suffering of others' actions and bodies the soul suffers some personal distress through the medium of speech'). Euripides echoes this argument in *Hippolytus*, where the Nurse complains that the care-giver suffers more than the patient:[6]

---

[6] The connection between the statement in *Breaths* and the words of the Nurse is noted in Wilamowitz' commentary on *Hippolytus ad loc*. Another parallel can be found in the *Dissoi Logoi* (DK 90 1 [3]). For more on this topos, see Jouanna's commentary on *Breaths ad loc*. (127–128).

κρεῖσσον δὲ νοσεῖν ἢ θεραπεύειν·
τὸ μέν ἐστιν ἁπλοῦν, τῷ δὲ συνάπτει
λύπη τε φρενῶν χερσίν τε πόνος.   (186–188)

It is better to be sick than to provide care for the sick:
For the former is a single issue, but in the latter case
pain of the mind and labor with the hands combine.

As much as this line of thinking may give us clues into Greek theory on the function of tragedy in society, characters within a tragedy would seem to have rather mixed feelings about the perspective on suffering espoused by the author of *Breaths*. Tragic figures spend impressive amounts of time focusing on and expressing their own suffering; the dying bemoan their loss of reputation and their pain, the surviving bemoan their own future in the absence of the fallen hero or heroine. Nonetheless, along with the expressions of suffering, there are usually attempts at healing and survival: both those who suffer and those who observe the suffering of others attempt to find remedies for the pain of living and the seeming inevitability of death.

This project is an exploration of Greek beliefs about suffering and the technology of healing in the fifth century BCE. It examines Greek explanations for the existence of suffering, the behavior of those who suffer, and the methods devised by humans to cope with suffering. The analysis focuses on aspects of suffering and healing in two corpora of fifth-century literature, the works of Euripides and of the Hippocratic writers, although it inevitably draws on material from other authors of the period as well. In this study, I argue that Euripidean tragedy, in its representations of the body in pain, also draws heavily upon ideas and images from the world of medicine. At the same time, I suggest that medicine and tragedy in the fifth century are drawing upon a common stock of ideas in Greek culture about the role of physical suffering and the nature of healing. Thus, by comparing and contrasting the ideas found in medicine and tragedy, I hope to illuminate patterns of thought that inform classical Greek views of disease, health and suffering.

Much of what I will say about medicine in the classical period has been well studied by other scholars. However, until recently—and with some important exceptions—such research has remained fairly isolated: while historians of medicine may have pointed to parallels in the literature of other genres, many have been more interested in Greek medicine's role in the development of Western medical thought than in placing Greek medicine in its own cultural context. Thus, they have sought out what was perceived to be successful, rational and useful in Greek medicine without always recognizing the gap between the ancient world and our own and likewise without examining Greek medical texts on their own terms. At the same time, as Thomas notes in her recent book on Herodotus, it is historians of medicine who have more often been interested in finding parallels between medical writing and other areas of Greek literature;[7] by contrast, the medical texts have been underused by those scholars working on more canonical works of the fifth century. In recent years, however, both historians of medicine and scholars of Greek literature have begun to examine Greek medical writing with the aim of better understanding its relationship to—and influence on—other areas of Greek culture. Thus, scholars have begun to mine the gynecological treatises of the Hippocratic Corpus in their attempts to understand ancient Greek beliefs and attitudes about women's nature.[8] There are also several important works that analyze medical beliefs (both parallel and contrasting) as represented in the Hippocratic Corpus and the historians of the fifth century.[9] In this study, I attempt to show that reading Greek tragedy through the lens of Greek medical theory reveals important aspects of Greek beliefs about pain and the human ability to comprehend and cope with pain through the use of *technê*.[10]

Certainly scholarly work on tragedy and medicine has not been lacking. Much of the scholarship investigating medical themes in tragedy has either focused on the use of technical medical vocabulary in individual plays and authors or on metaphors for disease in particular tragedies that are not necessarily closely related to medical literature. To be sure, several important analyses have focused more broadly on the issue of Hippocratic influence on tragedy, or at least looked for evidence of awareness by tragic authors of positions taken by Hippocratic authors. Collinge (1962) suggests that tragic use of medical themes is in general 'patchy, arbitrary, non-patterned and subject to sporadic con-

---

[7] Thomas (2000) 22.

[8] A growing body of scholarship: see, e.g., Manuli (1980) and (1983), Hanson (1990), Dean-Jones (1994), King (1998).

[9] On Herodotus, see especially Lateiner (1986) and now Thomas (2000); on Thucydides, a vast literature on the plague of Athens, but for a larger thematic study, see the important work of Rechenauer (1991).

[10] This word will be of great importance in this work. I understand it as a field-specific, teachable body of knowledge.

ventions.'[11] He maintains that, among the three great tragedians, only
Sophocles shows some signs of detailed understanding of medical ideas
and procedures ('Sophocles was, medically, an insider');[12] by contrast,
he suggests that Euripides, while aware of contemporary medical theories, is 'interested but uncommitted, commenting but not partaking.'[13]
Jouanna (1987) surveys tragic and Hippocratic approaches to a number of issues, including descriptions and causes of plague (*loimos*), the
use of technical medical vocabulary and representations of pathology.
Jouanna argues that the tragedians' use of medical themes incorporates traditional literary portraits of disease and healing more often
than contemporary medical ideas.[14] Furthermore, even when tragedians do refer to possible rationalist explanations for disease, they do not
rely on these explanations exclusively: instead, tragedians blend traditional, contemporary and religious thinking about disease and healing
in their representations of these issues. Moreover, as he points out,
pathological scenes in tragedy often involve madness,[15] whereas madness is not a major topos in extant medical literature.[16] He posits two
types of influence, one direct, as demonstrated by Euripides fr. 917
Nauck-Snell,[17] which speaks clearly of rationalist medical practices of
the fifth century, and one indirect, in which tragedians draw on contemporary medical language or practices as metaphors for the experiences of their tragic characters. Nonetheless, even in the cases of what

---

[11] Collinge (1962) 44.

[12] Collinge (1962) 47.

[13] Collinge (1962) 45.

[14] So, for example, the plague in *Oedipus Tyrannus* affects the entire animate population, whether it be animal, vegetable or human, whereas in the Hippocratic Corpus,
plague is a *miasma* in the air (according to *Breaths* 6) that affects specific individuals or
regions (Jouanna 1987: 111–112).

[15] He is not alone in emphasizing the importance of madness in tragedy. Simon
(1978) draws heavily upon tragedy in his discussion of the history of psychiatry; Padel
(1992) and (1995) argues that 'madness is central to tragedy' (1992: 163); for a discussion
of Padel's contributions to this issue, see Gill (1996b). See also Guardasole (2000) 160–
230 for an analysis of the pathology of madness in tragedy, which includes discussion of
many Hippocratic parallels.

[16] This is not to say that medical writers fail to mention delirium or other types of
psychological disorders; Jouanna himself points to several examples in the Hippocratic
Corpus where psychological factors are clearly at work in the illness of the patient (1987:
121–122).

[17] ὅσοι δ' ἰατρεύειν καλῶς, / πρὸς τὰς διαίτας τῶν ἐνοικούντων πόλιν / τὴν γῆν ἰδόντας
τὰς νόσους σκοπεῖν χρεών ('However many heal well, / must consider the diseases
with regard to the regimen of those inhabiting the polis / after having looked at the
environment').

he terms direct influence, Jouanna maintains that the tragedians continue to differ appreciably from the medical writers. So, for example, although, as has often been noted, tragic portrayals of madness reflect the symptoms of epilepsy (the 'sacred disease') described in the Hippocratic treatise *On the Sacred Disease*, tragedians freely adapt these symptoms to the needs of the production. In Jouanna's view, it is traditional tragic imagery of disease and rivalry with other poets that is of most significance in tragic representations of medical issues, rather than an engagement with contemporary rationalist thinkers. He suggests there is some variation among the playwrights on this question: references to medical ideas in Aeschylus, he suggests, can be explained by the existence of popular conceptions about disease which are then taken over and elaborated by the medical writers themselves, whereas Euripides, with his oft-noted interest in the latest intellectual movements of his day and his interest in realism, shows a greater awareness of ideas being circulated among rationalist healers.

In her two closely related studies ([1992] and [1995]), Padel has provided important analyses of Greek metaphors for disease and suffering in a wide range of literature from the archaic and classical periods— although she is concerned to stress the concreteness of much of this imagery, arguing that the language used is often an expression of a felt reality rather than a metaphor for it. Less focused than many scholars on the issue of determining whether a specific usage in tragedy belongs to the realm of 'technical' or 'scientific' terminology, Padel underscores the similarity of Hippocratic imagery for disease and suffering to that found in other Greek literature. Thus, for example, Padel examines Greek views of 'innards' (*splanchna*), of motion in the body, of moisture, of possession, demonic and otherwise, in a variety of genres and argues for the commonalities among them.[18]

In part as a response to the analysis of Jouanna,[19] Guardasole (2000) has undertaken a comprehensive study of medical imagery and terminology in all three tragedians. Her approach focuses on examining parallels between passages of the Hippocratic Corpus and passages in tragedy, showing points of contact and discontinuity. She amply demon-

---

[18] My approach differs from Padel's in that she is mostly interested in noting images of disease that recur throughout many tragedies, whereas I am trying to trace medical themes that carry throughout individual plays or at least throughout significant portions thereof.

[19] See Guardasole (2000) 28–29.

strates that there is cross-fertilization in the terminology of illness used
by the two very different genres. Moreover, she re-examines the disease
of madness, so prominent in tragedy, with reference to medical theory.
Guardasole's book is a valuable resource because of its broad scope
and references to many different passages in tragedy and Hippocratic
treatises. Referring not only to Euripidean plays but also to fragments
of Euripides that touch upon medical topics, she argues that Euripides shows a marked interest in the argumentative aspects of contemporary medicine—that is, in the rhetoric, the ideological controversies, the
intellectual debates that characterize Hippocratic medicine (such as the
promotion of dietetic medicine with its emphasis on prevention, versus
other therapies that rely on healing diseases after they have taken hold);
she also stresses Euripides' fascination with the psychological effects of
disease.[20]

Several studies have been directed specifically at medical themes in
Euripides. Ferrini (1978) shows the close correspondence between the
symptoms described by the author of *On the Sacred Disease* and those suffered by many Euripidean heroes and heroines as they undergo attacks
of disease, whether reported by messengers or depicted on stage. Ferrini argues that the many medical details provided by Euripides are
evidence of Euripidean 'realism.' He stresses Euripides' interest in the
physical manifestations of psychological illness, which also receive some
consideration in the Hippocratic Corpus. However, Ferrini focuses his
attention on the specific scenes in which characters go mad or become
ill; he does not examine how medical issues work themselves into the
fabric of an entire text. Smith (1967) provides an important foundation
for the study of the disease theme in *Orestes*, a play that has received
much attention because of its portrait of Orestes' Fury-driven madness;
rather than concentrating on only the 'sickness scene,' Smith shows
how the disease theme permeates the entire play. Most recently, Craik
(2001a) has investigated references to medical terms and healing strategies in Euripides; she argues that Euripides does show 'general famil-
iarity with many medical ideas,'[21] but that his use of medical ideas is a
complex blend of the technical and metaphorical. She maintains that
references in *Hippolytus* and a more widespread Euripidean interest in

---

[20] Guardasole (2000) 76–86. Although Guardasole does carry out extensive analyses
of some plays or scenes, she, like Padel, focuses more on imagery and terminology than
on what I will argue are themes sustained throughout a given play.

[21] Craik (2001a) 81 (in abstract).

the joints of the human body suggest that he may have had actual knowledge of the Hippocratic treatises *Breaths* and *Articulations* (also known as *Joints*). However, she argues, because 'the aims of medical writers and dramatists are fundamentally different ... verbal similarities can be deceptive.'[22]

In this study, rather than focusing on individual instances of medical vocabulary being employed in tragedy or analyzing various 'pathological scenes' in isolation, I intend to investigate broader patterns of engagement by Euripides in issues of disease and healing by examining a number of Euripidean tragedies through the lens of ancient medical theory. In so doing, I try to illuminate patterns of thinking shared by Greeks in the fifth century as they struggled to cope with pain, suffering, and disease. I contend that medical themes are more integrated into the work of Euripides than scholars have hitherto noticed. This, I suggest, is because of the position of medicine in Greek thinking in the late fifth century. In this period of intellectual and political ferment, the question of the limits and strengths of human intelligence took center stage, and the nature of *technê* found an important position in that discussion. Medicine, I suggest, had come to be seen as the human *technê* that best represented the successes and failures of human attempts to control the forces of nature. Thus, as we will see in greater detail in Part I, beginning with the poetry of Solon, it is medical *technê* that takes the capstone position in lists of technological endeavors. Its role in fifth-century thinking is epitomized by its significant placement in the second stasimon of Sophocles' *Antigone*, the so-called Ode to Man (332–375). Here, the human being is represented as something wondrous and strange, capable of overcoming many natural barriers through the application of technological skills. The list moves from navigation to agriculture to hunting, to the arts of speech and governance and protection against the elements. Finally, in the second strophe, the Chorus sing of how the human is resourceful in every way (παντόπορος, 360), yet it must admit that there are limits: without skills, the human cannot control nature, and he has no way to overcome death. Surprisingly, the strophe does not end here, but adds that humans have invented medicine as a means of escaping disease: νόσων δ' ἀμηχάνων φυγὰς / συμπέφρασται (363–364: 'but he has contrived escapes from uncontrollable diseases'). Death cannot be defeated, perhaps, but the diseases

---

[22] Craik (2001a) 86.

that lead to death can be controlled by medicine. These clever human skills can lead to good or ill, the chorus sing at the beginning of the second antistrophe: humans are in control of the *technai* they have devised, and they must apply these *technai* in morally sound ways. Euripides, likewise I argue, uses medical themes, strategies and metaphors in order to explore the human ability to cope with the hazards presented by nature and the gods, by *physis* and *tychê*.

I have chosen to focus on Euripides rather than on Aeschylus and Sophocles for different reasons. In the case of Aeschylus, as has been noted by other scholars, Greek rationalist medicine, as evidenced by the existence of the Hippocratic Corpus, is certainly under development during the poet's lifetime; however, from a methodological point of view, it is difficult to be sure that he would have been aware of arguments set forth in the writings of the Corpus itself, since most of these were composed after his death.[23] The works of Sophocles, of course, are not subject to such constraints; however, medical themes in Sophocles have already received some scholarly attention.[24] Furthermore, scholars have generally been receptive to seeing connections between Sophocles

---

[23] The study of medical vocabulary in Aeschylean tragedy is well-represented by Dumortier's work (1935). However, critics of Dumortier have appropriately pointed out that he pushes the connections between Aeschylus and the Hippocratic Corpus too hard (cf. Collinge [1962] 53 n. 1 and Guardasole [2000] 30–32); more recent scholarly discussions of medical issues in Aeschylus argue that his use of medical language and situations is drawn from popular contemporary usages and from his poetic predecessors: cf. Jouanna (1987) and Cordes (1994) 33–35. Recently, in her 1998 edition of *Places in Man*, Craik has argued that this treatise may be one of the earliest that we possess and dates it to the first half of the fifth century; if she is right, the ideas present in this text (with its emphasis on two humors, bile and phlegm, and its 'somewhat primitive' techniques [18]) would perhaps have been known to Aeschylus. The use of cautery and the idea of health as derived from the equilibrium of forces in the body, both prominent in *Places in Man*, were certainly known in Aeschylus' time. On the problem of the dating of the Hippocratic Corpus and the consequences for our understanding of Aeschylus's references to medicine, see now Guardasole (2000) 29–34. For an overview of the Hippocratic treatises and current scholarly opinion about their dates, see Appendix 3 in Jouanna (1999) 371–416.

[24] Disease themes in Sophocles have received some attention in discussions particularly of *Oedipus Tyrannus*, *Aias* and *Philoctetes*: On disease themes in Sophocles, with little focus on links to medical literature, see, e.g., Simpson (1969) and Ryzman (1992). Wilson (1941), Biggs (1966) and Worman (2000) argue for Sophoclean engagement with contemporary medical issues; Worman in particular has made some interesting remarks about parallel approaches to medical issues in the Hippocratic Corpus and in *Philoctetes*. Knox (1957) makes a direct connection between medical literature and *Oedipus Tyrannus*, arguing that Sophocles' portrait of Oedipus is in part modeled on the images of the rationalist healer found in the Hippocratic Corpus.

and medicine, perhaps in part because of Sophocles' biography: he is said to have played an important role in the introduction of the cult of Asclepius to Athens.[25] By contrast, while the relationship of Euripides to Greek medicine, as the brief review of scholarship above suggests, has not been overlooked, it has, as I intend to demonstrate, been underestimated.

In Part I of this study, I investigate the complex image of the healer in the literature of the fifth century, isolating two predominant images of the healer. On the one hand, there is the healer who cannot heal himself, exemplifying the limits of human intelligence, and, on the other, there is the healer who participates in the myth of progress so often rehearsed in the literature of the classical period and who, moreover, often takes pride of place as evidence of humans' ability to control nature and human destiny. I demonstrate how the largely optimistic portrait of the healer, particularly as represented in myths of progress, is manipulated within the texts of the medical writers themselves. I then explore the image of the healer in several works of Euripides and argue that for Euripides, the healing figure is more likely to be either incompetent or dangerous than a symbol of human progress. Thus, a contrast develops between the confident and authoritative view of the doctor's ability to diagnose and prognosticate that is found in the Hippocratic Corpus and the more skeptical attitude that evolves in tragedy. In Part II, I discuss Hippocratic ideas on disease causation and investigate the remedial strategies employed by healers whose techniques are described in the Hippocratic Corpus; thereafter, I demonstrate how these theories and strategies are likewise operative in Euripidean drama. Here again, a contrast emerges between the theories of cause and cure most often advocated by the medical writers and the ideas presented by the characters in tragic drama, even though these characters reveal an awareness of the medical recommendations.

My analysis does not assume an intimate knowledge of medical treatises on the part of the tragedians. Nevertheless, even though I cannot—and do not—claim that Euripides or his fellow tragedians studied medicine or read medical literature, it is also very likely that by the late fifth century, Athenian citizens would have some general knowledge of these theories because of the nature of medical practice

---

[25] Sources for this story include Philostratus *vita Apoll.* 3.17; Plut. *Numa* 4.6; *Etymologicum Magnum s.v.* δεξίων; see discussion in Guardasole (2000) 59–62; for the history of the shrine, see Aleshire (1989) 7–20.

in this period:[26] as Lloyd, Jouanna and others have stressed, the healing profession, like many others in the Greek world, was a competitive
one, and rationalist healers would no doubt have had opportunities to
declaim before Athenian audiences, whether they were competing to be
'state physicians' or merely looking for customers. On such occasions,
the healers would provide the citizens of Athens with access to rationalist medical theories; at the same time, they would have to use rhetoric
that would appeal to the public, and hence they would adopt and
manipulate traditional ideas about disease and healing. The boundaries between medicine, sophistry, philosophy, history and other intellectual movements were also quite fluid; at the same time, members of
the medical profession, like the Athenian tragedians, may have tried to
appeal to an audience more diverse than the elite classes attracted to
the theories and strategies of the philosophers and sophists.[27] I would
suggest that we find shared cultural assumptions in both the medical and tragic genres—and it is my aim to foreground some of these
assumptions.[28]

    Finally, a word on terminology, texts and translations. On terminol-
ogy: I avoid for the most part the words doctor and physician because
these words suggest a view of who qualifies as a member of the medical profession that is too restrictive in the context of fifth-century society. As I have just indicated, the boundaries between different types
of healers—let alone different types of professions—do not have ana-
logues that are easily recognizable in modern Western societies. A wide
range of persons could lay claim to the status of *iatros*. While the writers of the Hippocratic Corpus hasten to separate themselves from the
charlatans mentioned by the author of *On the Sacred Disease*, they are no
less eager to dismiss those within their own rationalist ranks with whom
they disagree. Non-healers such as Euripides may have understood that
approaches to healing varied widely among healers, but they may not
have distinguished rationalist healers as *iatroi* while designating root-

---

[26] For an excellent discussion of the problems that arise in trying to locate allusions
to specific medical treatises in tragedy, see Craik (2001a), esp. 81–86.

[27] On rhetoric in medicine and the implications of the need of physicians to persuade their listeners, see Lloyd (1979); Jouanna (1999) 75–85; Nutton (1992).

[28] I also believe that the experience of disease itself is fairly universal; that is, at some
point in his or her life, almost everyone either suffers from disease or cares for a sick
person, and must decide what to do about the situation. The tragedians of the fifth
century may not have known much about rationalist medicine, but they surely had
some interest in the subject simply because of their own personal needs.

cutters or herb-sellers as something else entirely. This does not mean that no distinctions were made by the general public between different approaches to healing.[29] Furthermore, as scholars have shown and as this analysis will confirm, the healers represented in the Hippocratic Corpus may often dress traditional healing ideas in new language, but many of their theories remain closely connected to notions of disease and healing widespread in the ancient Greek world. The distinction between the true doctor and the false is not one easily made from this distance of time and space. Hence, in an attempt to avoid misleading nomenclature, I will generally use the more neutral word healer in my discussions here.

On the texts of the Hippocratic Corpus: in the text, I have used the most common English titles for the treatises; in the footnotes, I have generally used the Latin titles or abbreviations for brief citations. When quoting at length from the Corpus or discussing a treatise in detail, I have cited from modern editions of the treatises (when available) in preference to the Littré version. Unless otherwise stated, I have given citations of passages in the footnotes as they occur in the *Thesaurus Linguae Graecae* and/or in Maloney and Frohn (1986): these generally refer to the Littré edition.

On translations: all translations, unless otherwise noted, are my own. I have made no attempt at elegance but have instead tried to provide translations that are both fairly literal and at the same time intelligible.

---

[29] Note, for example, the two possible types of healers suggested by Heracles at *Trachiniae* 1000–1001: τίς γὰρ ἀοιδός, τίς ὁ χειροτέχνας / ἰατορίας, ὃς τάνδ' ἄτην / χωρὶς Ζηνὸς κατακλήσει; ('For who is the enchanter, who is the practitioner of healing, who will lull this destruction to sleep except for Zeus?') and cf. the remarks of Cordes (1994) 39 n. 30, who adduces *Aias* 581 as additional evidence for the idea that the Greeks made distinctions between magical and medical types of healing.

PART I

HEALERS AND THE HEROICS OF MEDICAL *TECHNÊ*

CHAPTER ONE

THE HEALING ART

a. *The Healer: Lively metaphor and lived reality*

The role of healer as represented in our literary sources from antiquity is diverse and changeable. The healer as a metaphor or metonym for authority, cleverness and/or skill (so prominent in the images drawn from scientific medicine today) is normal but rare in the literature of the archaic period[1]— such images are more likely to be supplied by other workers with technical skills, such as ship's captains, seers and singers.[2] By contrast, in the literature of the classical period, the figure of the healer occurs regularly, but the image becomes more elaborate, with both negative and positive resonances. Exactly why the image becomes both more complex and more frequent is cause only for speculation (especially given the limited evidence available for the archaic period), but I suspect there are a number of different factors involved: the increasing range of healing options available, from the traditional root-cutters and midwives to the healing dreams and hands of the god Asclepius to the wide range of self-consciously rationalistic healers represented in the Hippocratic Corpus; the self-advertisement of sophisticated healers using both written and oral forms of communication; and finally, developments in other areas of Greek culture, from sculpture and painting to athletic training to natural philosophy, that intersect with medical interests not only in the healthy functioning of the human body but also in concepts of professionalism. The analysis that follows will trace briefly the history of the healer's image in archaic literature and then explore the complexity of this image as it flourished in the fifth century. I will first examine healers represented in non-medical

---

[1] Hesiod is typical of much of extant archaic literature in that his work features no prominent discussion of healers at all; only the *iatromantis* Melampus receives notice (on whom see in text below). Cordes (1994: 18) argues that this lack results from Hesiod's pessimistic view of disease as a punishment for humankind.

[2] On metaphors and analogies drawn from those who possess technical skills, see Detienne and Vernant (1978) *passim*; for their discussion of healers, see 307–313.

literature and then turn to an investigation of healers as they portray themselves in the texts of the Hippocratic Corpus. I maintain that as healers themselves reach out to interact with other areas of Greek culture and make increasingly greater claims for the centrality and sophistication of the healing art, so, then, do those other areas respond with greater attention to the claims and ideas put forth by members of the healing 'profession.' While health and disease had surely always been a focus of the Greeks in any era, metaphors and images derived from healers and the healing arts became more complex as the healing arts developed new strategies and, perhaps more important, new rhetoric. Hence, by the late fifth century, as this analysis will demonstrate, healers and their theories play an important role in a wide range of literary venues, from comedy and tragedy to historiography to philosophy. A detailed examination of several Euripidean tragedies will serve as a proving ground for the truth of this argument.

Healers are mentioned in our earliest literary sources: Homer speaks in the *Iliad* of the *iatroi*-warriors Machaon and Podalirus, sons of Asclepius, who appear in the catalogue of ships as leaders of ships from Thessaly. Machaon is featured on various occasions, whereas Podalirus plays only a minor role (although it is likely that he had a more prominent part in the other poems of the cycle: both brothers appear in the *Iliu Persis*, for example). Machaon is not a member of the inner circle of Greek chieftains, but he is accorded respect and attention both by the poet and by the characters he portrays. The wounding of Machaon occasions special concern, because, as Idomeneus says to Nestor, a healer is a man worth many others (11.514). Healers seem to have been accorded respect in Homeric society, even if their roles in the *Iliad* are not so significant as those of seers or even singers. In the plague that takes place in Book 1 of the *Iliad*, it is a seer to whom the Greeks turn for answers, not a healer; and Patroclus and Achilles seem to be quite as expert at medicine as the characters named as healers. Indeed, healing skills seem to have been part of the traditional training of heroes, as attested by the myths of Chiron, wise centaur skilled in healing arts and instructor of youthful heroes. The *Iliad* thus depicts healing as both an area of specialization and as a skill necessarily possessed by warrior chiefs at the highest levels of society.[3]

---

[3] On Podalirus, see Edelstein and Edelstein (1998) vol. II, 10–17. On the significance of Machaon and on the conception of healers in the *Iliad*, see Cordes (1994) 12–16.

In *Odyssey* 17, we are given another picture of the healer, and one which is to some extent reflected in our later sources: when Odysseus finally reaches home on Ithaca and enters his household disguised as a beggar, he is abused by the evil suitor Antinous, who is then rebuked by the swineherd Eumaeus:

> Ἀντίνο᾽, οὐ μὲν καλὰ καὶ ἐσθλὸς ἐὼν ἀγορεύεις·
> τίς γὰρ δὴ ξεῖνον καλεῖ ἄλλοθεν αὐτὸς ἐπελθὼν
> ἄλλον γ᾽, εἰ μὴ τῶν οἳ δημιοέργοι ἔασι,
> μάντιν ἢ ἰητῆρα κακῶν ἢ τέκτονα δούρων
> ἢ καὶ θέσπιν ἀοιδόν, ὅ κεν τέρπῃσιν ἀείδων;
> οὗτοι γὰρ κλητοί γε βροτῶν ἐπ᾽ ἀπείρονα γαῖαν·
> πτωχὸν δ᾽ οὐκ ἄν τις καλέοι τρύξοντα ἓ αὐτόν.　　　　(381–387)

> Antinoos, although you are noble, you do not speak well:
> for who calls another stranger from elsewhere, going himself,
> unless he is one of the workers for the people,
> a seer or a healer of ills or a fashioner of wood
> or a divine singer, who takes delight in song?
> For these are the summoned of mortals on the boundless earth;
> but someone would not summon a beggar who would eat up what
>   he has.

Here, healers are placed in the category of the *dêmioergoi*, the workers for the people, a group which also includes seers, singers and woodworkers, and they seem to be an itinerant group, moving around 'on call' (*klêtoi*) from household to household and welcomed because they serve a valuable function. Thus, the Homeric poems give us two different views of the healing profession: the Iliadic view, in which elite warriors like Machaon and Podalirus practice healing for no material reward, and the Odyssean one, in which healers are removed from the category of the elite and placed into the ranks of professional workers. It may well be that such a two-tiered system of healers existed throughout antiquity, the one an elite group practicing medicine as a benefaction for others and the other a professional group, often itinerant, practicing their craft for a fee.[4] On the other hand, the distinction between healers in the two poems can also be explained by the social situations described therein: the war society of the *Iliad* is dominated by the members of the elite who must at the same time fend for themselves, whereas the domestic situation of the *Odyssey* reveals the specialists who would be available on the home front.[5]

---

[4] See Horstmanshoff (1990) 188–196.
[5] See Cordes (1994) 17 n. 13.

As already mentioned, images of authority in archaic literature rest largely with kings or warriors, and, among persons with a particular skill (*technê*), ship-captains, seers and charioteers.[6] Many of these skill-ful persons figure either actually or metaphorically as representatives of *mêtis*. As Detienne and Vernant (1978) have shown, *mêtis* ('cunning intelligence') has a long and important history among Greek 'mental categories,' and a wide variety of human skills are used to illustrate the virtues and deficits of this quality. In the complex tale of *technê* told in the *Odyssey*, the magical arts of Circe, for example, demonstrate the negative potential of *technê*, while Odysseus, the master craftsman, uses *technê* to outwit both monsters and monstrous human beings. But, in Homer, *technê*, whether a sign of wiliness or an indicator of human competence, is generally unfailing.[7] However, the aspects of deceitful-ness and wiliness that are firmly attached to figures possessing *mêtis* do not typify those specified as healers in Homer, where the healer, if men-tioned at all, is only mentioned as welcome and valuable.[8]

By contrast, in the literature of the seventh century, authors begin to refer to the limitations of the medical art. Solon provides some of the scanty testimony for these less optimistic images of healers when he lists a variety of professions in fragment 13 West. The list seems to be roughly organized on a scale that begins with the less elite (sea-merchants, then farmers) and moves to more elite (poets, seers). Healers are placed just before seers at the very end and given more verses than

---

[6] Weaving also supplies an image of authoritative skill for women, but it is usually associated with deceit and trickery, as well.

[7] On the complexities of *technê* in Homer, see Roochnik (1996) 18–26; Roochnik argues that the prevalent meaning of *technê* in the Homeric poems refers to a skill which is productive (as in woodworking or smithing), and that this is why healers are not mentioned in the context of *technê*, but rather only as *dêmiourgoi*: healers, like seers and poets, do not produce anything. At the same time, Roochnik demonstrates that the term *technê* has 'potential latent for expansion,' given its associations with guile and craftiness both in Homer and Hesiod (25).

[8] This is not true of one aspect of the medical art, however: the use of *pharmaka*, which are substances which can both heal and harm, is problematic—cf., e.g., Helen's use of *pharmaka* in *Odyssey* 4 and the associations of *pharmaka* with mystery and magic elsewhere in the *Odyssey* (such as the wily Odysseus' use of the plant *môly* [described at 10.304]). However, magical potions are in some ways distinct from the remedies of the *iatroi* in the world of the epic; they are taken internally, whereas the remedies of *iatroi* and other healers mentioned in Homer are external salves. Helen's use of *nêpenthê* (*Odyssey* 4.221) to purge/prevent emotional distress is an interesting case which may show the influence of Egyptian medical knowledge in this period—but Helen is not an *iatra*, nor is her drug said to heal anything here, even though it enables a certain kind of emotional healing. See the detailed analysis of *nêpenthê* in Lorenz (1990) 31–38.

any of the other groups, suggesting their great importance in Solon's scheme. Yet, these Solonian healers cannot be said to have predictable, reliable success rates; indeed, although the work of the healer is placed in the category of *technê*, healers are as subject to chance and misfortune in the course of their duties as any other mortal being. Furthermore, confidence in their ability to heal rests more on what seems to be a miraculous healing touch than on the use of gentle remedies.

πολλάκι δ' ἐξ ὀλίγης ὀδύνης μέγα γίγνεται ἄλγος,
    κοὐκ ἄν τις λύσαιτ' ἤπια φάρμακα δούς·
τὸν δὲ κακαῖς νούσοισι κυκώμενον ἀργαλέαις τε
    ἁψάμενος χειροῖν αἶψα τίθησ' ὑγιῆ.   (59–62)

Often from a small pain great pain arises,
    and someone could not relieve it having given soothing drugs:
but a person distressed by evil and painful diseases
    having touched him with his hands he straightaway makes healthy.

The simple touch of a hand can cure one man right away, while the skilled application of 'soothing drugs' may have no impact at all.[9] Throughout this poem, Solon suggests that it is simply impartial Moira which brings good or bad to the individual and indicates that humans have little control over aspects of health and wealth in their own lives.[10]

Technai can fail, as Solon informs us (and, to be sure, *technê* may always have been a poor substitute for the spontaneous abundance of the Golden Age that is represented in Hesiod [*Works and Days* 109–126]). However, if healers in Solon fail, it is not because they themselves are morally worse than other humans or because their *technê* is inherently problematic. Instead, they fail because they exemplify the human inability to control completely the workings of nature.

---

[9] Here I part company with Cordes' excellent discussion of medical issues in Solon ([1994] 19–23). He asserts forcefully that there is no suggestion of the miraculous in the touch here, but rather that Solon probably refers to surgical measures such as cutting, burning, treatment of wounds, bone-setting, etc (21). The problem with his interpretation, in my opinion, is Solon's use of the word αἶψα, 'straightaway.' The idea of surgical methods curing problems immediately seems inherently unrealistic, and the interpretation also accords ill with Solon's pessimistic view of the human ability to overcome problems with *technê* expressed in the poem.

[10] As Roochnik (1996: 31) writes, Solon's definition of *technê* is 'use- or value-neutral and cannot in itself bring happiness.' However, despite his apparent skepticism over the reliability of medical methods, Solon is said to have tried to encourage the immigration of craftspeople such as healers to Attica in an effort to upgrade services available: as Plutarch reports in his *Life of Solon*, Solon urged itinerants 'to change residence for the sake of *technê*' (μετοικίζεσθαι ἐπὶ τέχνῃ, 24.4).

In the classical period, the figure of the healer begins to appear in literary efforts with increasing frequency. The very fact that literature from this era has survived in greater amounts may account for this fact, yet, as I will argue, developments within the field of medicine itself—including increased self-advertisement—did not escape the notice of the public at large. These developments include not only the rise of Hippocratic medicine, but also a perceptible growth of interest in the cult of the healing god Asclepius. Indeed, Asclepius is represented as the one healer whose *technê* is unfailing, if he chooses to apply it. In *Pythian* 3, Pindar describes the infallibility of the healing god Asclepius in whatever method he chooses, whether it be drugs or incantations or surgery:

> τοὺς μὲν ὦν, ὅσσοι μόλον αὐτοφύτων
> ἑλκέων ξυνάονες, ἢ πολιῷ χαλκῷ μέλη τετρωμένοι
> ἢ χερμάδι τηλεβόλῳ,
> ἢ θερινῷ πυρὶ περθόμενοι δέμας ἢ χειμῶνι, λύσαις ἄλλον ἀλλοίων ἀχέων
> ἔξαγεν, τοὺς μὲν μαλακαῖς ἐπαοιδαῖς ἀμφέπων,
> τοὺς δὲ προσανέα πίνοντας, ἢ γυίοις περάπτων πάντοθεν
> φάρμακα, τοὺς δὲ τομαῖς ἔστασεν ὀρθούς.   (47–53)

Of those, however many came suffering from natural
sores, or wounded in their limbs by grey bronze
or by stone hurled from afar
or wasting away in their bodies from summer's heat or from cold,
    loosening different ones from different pains
he delivered them, tending some with gentle incantations,
others drinking soothing drinks, or applying to their limbs on all sides
drugs, and others he set right by cutting.

Of course, it should be noted that this poem, which celebrates Asclepius' abilities to heal, also provides a warning: for Pindar tells us how Asclepius, having been given a bribe, used his powers to bring a dead man back to life; in response, Zeus killed Asclepius with a thunderbolt. This story shows us both the extraordinary power accorded to the healing art, but also suggests some suspicion regarding the motivations of its practitioners: they are corruptible, greedy for gain. By contrast, in *Pythian* 4, the image of the healer is unambiguously positive: in this ode, Pindar praises the leadership capacity of Arcesilaus by calling him an ἰατὴρ ἐπικαιρότατος ('a healer with a most excellent sense of timing,' 271) who knows how to use gentle methods to heal a wound.[11] Hence,

---

[11] Cordes (1994: 26) points out that this is the first time in extant literature that a political leader is likened to a healer.

Pindar's poetry suggests two issues at work with regard to the images of
healers in Greek society: the healing art and those who practice it well
are praiseworthy, yet at the same time healers, since they must practice a trade and seek payment in order to make their living, are not
motivated by the search for honor and respect that is the reward for
excellence among the elite. Medicine is not able to bring the rewards
that Pindar's song can, nor does the skill of the healer bring the great
satisfaction that more intangible qualities provided by the Muses do: as
Pindar writes in *Nemean* 4,

> ἄριστος εὐφροσύνα πόνων κεκριμένων ἰατρός· αἱ δὲ σοφαὶ
> Μοισᾶν θύγατρες ἀοιδαὶ θέλξαν νιν ἁπτόμεναι.
> οὐδὲ θερμὸν ὕδωρ τόσον γε μαλθακὰ τεύχει
> γυῖα, τόσσον εὐλογία φόρμιγγι συνάορος.   (1–4)

> Good cheer is the best healer when contests have been ended; the wise
> daughters of the Muses, songs, having taken hold, soothe him.
> Nor does warm water put his limbs at ease
> as much as praise in accompaniment with the lyre.

Among the issues addressed thus far, two deserve further attention: first,
what was the social status accorded to healers in the archaic and classical periods? And, second, what was the nature of the *technê* practiced by
the healers that rendered them not only valuable as healers but also as
metaphors for human accomplishment and failure? The two issues of
status and *technê* are in fact very much intertwined, but nonetheless let
us defer a detailed analysis of the *technê* itself for the moment. As noted
above, healers are classified among the elite in the *Iliad*, but as *dêmioergoi*
in the *Odyssey*. The *dêmioergoi* are clearly important to the community—
because they provide specialized services—but at the same time they
are in a different category than the heroes who risk their lives in the
pursuit of *aretê* (excellence). Often itinerant, making their living at the
behest of others' demands, they are free men practicing a trade, but
they do not own land, possession of which was a fundamental dividing line in both archaic and classical Greek society.[12] Having wealth as
a matter of birth, handed down from one's ancestors, is acceptable in
the Greek aristocratic value system, but working to gain wealth by the
labor of one's hands is denigrated. Elites might act to benefit others at
some cost to themselves, but that is in part because they were in posi-

---

[12] On the possession of land and its importance in Greek society, see Burford
(1993) esp. 66–95; but note also the removal of land-ownership as a qualification for
citizenship in democratic Athens (cf. Pericles at Thucydides 2.37.1).

tions of power and could afford to do so—indeed, in Athens at least, liturgies performed by the elite demonstrated at the same time their high status and their willingness to support the interests of the democratic state; through benefiting the state, they achieved honor (*timê*). Craftsmen, by contrast, were expected to be motivated primarily by the need to work rather than by the desire for *timê*.[13] The practitioners of *technê* were subject to the disdain of the elite since they were deprived of manly pursuits such as exercise and were perceived to have little time to participate in the larger demands of civic life; they often worked, as Xenophon in *Oeconomicus* 4.3 points out, in poor conditions, indoors all day. The attitude that devalues the work of the *technitês*, the craftsman, in comparison to the warrior or citizen elite is apparent not only in Homer and Pindar but also in numerous other writers; it is abundantly clear in the works of elitist writers such as Plato, Xenophon and Aristotle, who feature criticism of *technitai* (other terms include *cheironax* and *cheirotechnês*, meaning 'handworker' with obvious emphasis on the *cheir*, the hand) in their dismissive discussions of *banausia* (servile or manual labor, labor at the behest of others).[14] Only the manual labor of the self-sufficient country farmer, the *autourgos* who owns a small bit of property, regularly wins praise in our literary sources. Indeed, the evidence suggests that it was considered far better to be even a poor *autourgos* than an itinerant healer or some pottery painter settled in a workshop in Athens.[15] Later sources continue to show us this ambivalence in evaluating technicians: while all seem to agree that *technê* itself provides important benefits for humanity, we continue to find writers expressing reservations over the status of the technicians themselves. Plutarch writes in his *Life of Pericles*:

πολλάκις δὲ καὶ τοὐναντίον χαίροντες τῷ ἔργῳ τοῦ δημιουργοῦ καταφρο-
νοῦμεν ... καὶ οὐδεὶς εὐφυὴς νέος ἢ τὸν ἐν Πίσῃ θεασάμενος Δία γενέσθαι
Φειδίας ἐπεθύμησεν, ἢ τὴν Ἥραν τὴν ἐν Ἄργει Πολύκλειτος, οὐδ᾿ Ἀνα-
κρέων ἢ Φιλήμων ἢ Ἀρχίλοχος ἡσθεὶς αὐτῶν τοῖς ποιήμασιν.   (1.4–2.1)

---

[13] Of course, as early as Hesiod, we hear of rivalry between potters as well as poets (*Works and Days* 25–26). The agonistic element in Greek culture plays a powerful role in those who practice *technai*; there is plenty of evidence for this in the medical arena, well discussed in Lloyd (1987) 97–100.

[14] On the status of craftsmen and the issue of *banausia*, see, among others, Burford (1972) 28–36; on the rhetoric involving 'servile' status in Athenian society, see Ober (1989) 272–277; finally, on the rhetoric of *banausia* in Plato, see Nightingale (1995) 55–59.

[15] On the value of *autourgoi*, see esp. Xenophon, *Oec.* 4.2–3.

On the contrary, often we look down upon the craftsman while delight-
ing in his work … No gifted young man, having seen the Zeus at
Olympia or the Hera at Argos, ever actually wanted to be Phidias or
Polyclitus nor to be Anacreon or Philemon or Archilochus, though taking pleasure in their songs.

At the same time, as Ellen Wood emphasizes, it is important to distinguish 'contempt for servility … from a disdain for labour.'[16] Hard work
is certainly valued in Greek society: even our most elitist writers do
not honor idleness. Rather, they reserve their highest praise for those
who labor only for themselves. Aristotle's argument at *Politics* 1277b5–7
demonstrates that it is not labor per se, but rather in whose interest
and towards which goal the labor is directed that creates problems.[17]
Moreover, as I will discuss further below, the application of technology,
usually associated with the use of the hands, is regarded as essential in
the course of human progress. Hence, a tension arises over the status of
the *technitai*: their work is valuable and adds to the well being of society,
yet at the same time they are wage-earners who work with their hands.
Evidence suggests that most healers were free men, but not members of
the aristocracy.[18] Those few healers who were members of the elite class
probably performed their work as a type of benefaction and so did not
earn the disdain of their fellow elite.[19] Some healers were clearly in high
demand and earned not only wealth but respect. Herodotus tells us the
story of Democedes, a Greek healer of some renown in the late sixth
century, who was captured by the Persians but who was set free and
hired by the Persian King Darius when his profession was discovered
(3.125–137). The story of Democedes suggests that a number of healers active in the sixth century received public recognition—and even
public compensation.[20]

By Plato's time, the healer has become a regular feature of discourse,
invoked frequently in Plato's dialogues as a model of knowledgeable,
skilled authority.[21] Yet the *iatros* figure in Plato is a complex one with

---

[16] Wood (1988) 137.
[17] On the attitudes of Aristotle and Plato towards 'banausic' occupations, see Nightingale (1995) 55–59.
[18] On the controversial issue of the slave healers mentioned in Plato's *Laws*, see
Nightingale (1999) 117–120.
[19] See Horstmanshoff (1990) 193–197.
[20] On the tradition of 'state' physicians in Greece, see Cohn-Haft (1956) and Jouanna
(1999) 76–80.
[21] Along with shoemakers, carpenters, pilots, and cooks, healers exemplify practitioners of a *technê* in Plato. Salkever (1994) argues that the concept of *technê* pro-

both positive and negative resonances; the issue of his social status is
not always allied with the issue of his social value. So, for example,
Callicles in *Gorgias* finds it offensive and annoying that Socrates keeps
introducing technicians, such as shoemakers and fullers and cooks and
doctors into his arguments (491a1–3), and he is not alone among Plato's
interlocutors in finding such characters inappropriate to sophisticated
speech. At the same time, we find Plato's most developed portrait of
a healer, the *iatros* Eryximachus in *Symposium*, participating fully in the
elite pastime of the symposium. Eryximachus may be a rather foolish
figure, appearing more pompous than authoritative, and he fails to provide a better explanation of love than the comedian Aristophanes, but
he is at least present and apparently accepted at an elite event.[22] Furthermore, in the *Laws*, Plato envisions an idealized *iatros*, who, understanding the link between the body and the soul, tends to the condition of both; this *iatros*, who attends to free men, is contrasted with the
iatros of slaves, who merely attends to the physical needs of his patients
and tells them what to do, rather than working with them to achieve a
unified mental and physical health (720a2-e5). Indeed, most of Plato's
healers are ultimately no match for his philosophers, attending as they
do only to the health of the body and not to the health of the soul; in
Plato's view, they are better compared to statesmen or lawgivers than
to philosophers. Thus, their role is to rule their patients with authority,
rather than to bring to birth the wisdom of the patient (to use the mid-
wife imagery employed by Socrates in *Symposium*). Plato is critical of the
healers of his day whom he accuses of pampering patients, prolonging
the lives of more or less useless people and using newfangled methods
such as control of regimen rather than more traditional harsh remedies

---

vides a solid source of authority readily intelligible to Plato's audience; thus, the Pla-
tonic Socrates often refers to *technê* when setting up his arguments because the ideas
expressed by the term *technê* are more accessible to his interlocutors than his rather
novel appeals to abstract notions of justice, *aretê*, and *to kalon*; the notion of *technê* thus
provides a good starting point for the process of *elenchos*. Cf. also Lidz (1995) for the
importance of the medical model in Plato's ethics.

[22] Edelstein (1967), against the prevailing views of scholarship, argues that Eryximachus should be taken quite seriously. While he makes a number of useful observations (especially concerning Eryximachus' role as a catalyst for the topos and progress
of the conversation [164]), his argument that Plato's portrait of this *iatros* and his recommendations is a largely complimentary one seems problematic to me, given how
the other characters tend to tease him and given his attack of hiccups. On medical
aspects of the speeches of Eryximachus and Aristophanes (noting in particular how
Aristophanes' speech responds to that of Eryximachus), see Craik (2001b).

(*Republic* 3.404a1–410a6).[23] As Cordes suggests, in some of Plato's works, the very existence of the medical art is a sign of luxurious living and thus an 'Indiz menschlicher Dekadenz'—a sign of decline and corruption from an earlier stage of human existence when humans did not need to be pampered.[24]

Defining the status of a healer is further complicated by the problem of figuring out who fits into the category. There are figures called *iatromanteis*, 'healer-seers' who perform various healing acts: a famous example is the *iatromantis* Melampus, mentioned in fragments of the poet Hesiod (fr. 37 Merkelbach-West), who cured the daughters of Proteus of madness. Then there are purifiers (*kathartai*) with complex professional qualifications: perhaps the most well-known of these is the Presocratic philosopher Empedocles, who according to Diogenes Laertius wrote an *Iatrikos Logos* of 600 verses.[25] In Empedocles' poem entitled *Katharmoi* (*Purifications*), he claimed to the citizens of Acragas that he was a healer of great distinction: his methods, to the extent that we can discern them, seem to involve ritual purifications and words. In fragment 112, which gives the opening lines of the poem, he represents himself as divine and states that men and women follow him, some seeking words of prophecy, while others ἐπὶ νούσων / παντοίων ἐπύθοντο κλύειν εὐηκέα βάξιν (9–10: 'were seeking to hear a healing utterance against diseases of every kind'). Another example is the Cretan Epimenides, who was brought to Athens in the late sixth century to cure a plague: he did so by performing a propitiatory sacrificial ritual.[26]

---

[23] As Horstmanhoff (1990) notes in his discussion of the ambiguous status of healers, healers in the elite group refused pay for services and attempted to ally their profession with the noble art of philosophy, '[y]et medicine was never able to find a respectable place among the *artes liberales*, even by connecting up with philosophy which stood higher than the *artes liberales*' (195).

[24] Cordes (1994) 190, and on the complex image of the *iatros* in Plato, 138–169.

[25] Cf. Diog. Laert. 8.77 (= DK31 A1); the poem is not accepted as authentic: see Kirk, Raven, Schofield (1983) 283 n. 1.

[26] For an account of Epimenides in Athens, see Diog. Laert. 1.110 (= DK3 A1). On *iatromanteis* and Epimenides in particular, see Dodds (1951) 140–146 and on *iatromanteis* and *kathartai* see Hoessly (2001) 173–197.

b. Technê *and* Technitai *in the Hippocratic Corpus*

The distinctions between religious and naturalistic methods of healing
were still being worked out in the classical period—although I should
add that arguments over such distinctions continued for centuries. Even
those who were attended by *iatroi* working in the rationalist tradition (as
represented in the Hippocratic Corpus) were probably much less prone
than twentieth century scholars to make distinctions between religion,
magic, and secular medicine. Indeed, the same patient might sleep in
the sanctuary of Asclepius at Epidaurus, make use of herbs gathered in
the dark of the moon while chanting spells and invoking Hecate, and
go to a healer in pursuit of some rationalist dietary or pharmacological cure. To the average Greek of this period, all of these approaches
were merely different routes to the same end: the restoration of their
health. Health was their primary concern.[27] But the practitioners of
these trades had a different point of view: they had to convince people that their method worked.[28] And the medical writers of the Hippocratic Corpus set out to show through theory and argument and
occasionally experiment why their method was the most likely to succeed. In treatises (some perhaps delivered in public) such as *On Ancient
Medicine* and *The Art*, rationalist healers argued that the art of medicine
deserved its own name, its own definition, and was indeed worthy of
the designation *iatrikê technê*.[29] At the same time, these healers were trying to claim new territory and new authority for themselves not only
by turning to ideas found in Presocratic and sophistic circles but also
by assimilating traditional cultural models and practices to their own
work. In a well-known example, the author of *Prognostic* appropriates
language traditionally referring to the work of prophets and poets when
he states that a physician must be able to 'announce without being told
the past, the present, and the future' (προλέγων ... τά τε παρέοντα καὶ

---

[27] On the medical marketplace model, see the various articles of Nutton (1985; 1992;
1995) and an account by King (1998) 100–113, with a nuanced critique of the use of this
idea in scholarship on the history of medicine.

[28] For a discussion of common perceptions of healers and medicine in classical
antiquity and on the importance of *logos* in the success of medical treatment, see Nutton
(1985).

[29] Indeed, some of the more theoretical of Hippocratic treatises, such as *The Art*, are
practically hymns to *technê*. As noted earlier (note 13), G.E.R. Lloyd has demonstrated
the competitive nature of Greek medicine and the importance of rhetoric and debate in
the construction of many medical treatments; see Lloyd (1979) and (1987). For the issue
of oral delivery, see Thomas (1993).

τὰ προγεγονότα καὶ τὰ μέλλοντα ἔσεσθαι, 1).[30] Moreover, the explanations of disease and treatment found in the Corpus, as will be discussed more thoroughly in Part II, often draw upon ideas with a long history in Greek thought, such as purification (*katharsis*)[31] and even pollution (*miasma*). Hence, by the late fifth century, it is clear on the one hand that to find acceptance among the public the rationalist *iatroi* must appeal to cultural norms; at the same time, they are also trying very hard to differentiate their etiologies of disease and methodologies of healing from that of seers and purifiers.[32] The author of the text *On the Sacred Disease* is scathing in his attacks on the purifiers and charlatans who claim that the 'sacred disease,' which is the traditional Greek name for epilepsy, is caused by an attack of the gods and thus can be cured by prayers, purifications and avoidance of certain substances that have a symbolic association with the disease.[33] Our author, stating confidently that the disease is not brought on by the gods, but is due to natural causes, criticizes those with a more traditional view:

> ἐμοὶ δὲ δοκέουσιν οἱ πρῶτοι τοῦτο τὸ νόσημα ἱρώσαντες τοιοῦτοι εἶναι ἄνθρωποι οἷοι καὶ νῦν εἰσι μάγοι τε καὶ καθάρται καὶ ἀγύρται καὶ ἀλαζόνες, ὁκόσοι προσποιέονται σφόδρα θεοσεβέες εἶναι καὶ πλέον τι εἰδέναι. οὗτοι τοίνυν παραμπεχόμενοι καὶ προβαλλόμενοι τὸ θεῖον τῆς ἀμηχανίης τοῦ μὴ ἔχειν ὅ τι προσενέγκατες ὠφελήσουσι καὶ ὡς μὴ κατάδηλοι ἔωσιν οὐδὲν ἐπιστάμενοι, ἱρὸν ἐνόμισαν τοῦτο τὸ πάθος εἶναι, καὶ λόγους ἐπιλέξαντες ἐπιτηδείους τὴν ἴησιν κατεστήσαντο ἐς τὸ ἀσφαλὲς σφίσιν αὐτοῖσι καθαρμοὺς προσφέροντες καὶ ἐπαοιδάς, ...   (1.10–12 Grensemann)

It seems to me that those who first called this disease sacred are men such as we now call witch-doctors and purifiers and quacks and charla-

---

[30] Cf. the prophet Calchas in *Iliad* 1.70, the poet Demodocus as described in *Odyssey* 8.491–498, and Hesiod and his Muses at *Theogony* 31–39. On the relationship between medicine and divination in this period, see Langholf (1990) 232ff. Langholf cautions, 'It must, however, be stated ... that such references to or vestiges of divination are by no means an outstanding feature of the Hippocratic collection. The references are scarce and the vestiges are not easily noted without scrutiny' (235). He goes on to write: 'Even though for the medical craftsmen of the Hippocratic collection there appears to have existed a relatively clear-cut distinction between medical prognosis and divination (the latter craft being practised by other craftsmen), large parts of the population seem to have been rather indifferent to such a distinction. This situation is well illustrated by the occasional reference to the *iatromantis*, "physician and seer," in sources outside of the Hippocratic collection' (235).

[31] For extensive discussion of the connections between religious and medical *katharsis*, see Hoessly (2001).

[32] A major theme of Lloyd's work; see Lloyd (1979), especially 15–29 and 86–98.

[33] For an extensive discussion of the rhetorical nature of *On the Sacred Disease*, see Laskaris (2002).

tans, all indeed who pretend to be reverent of the gods and to be especially knowledgeable in some way. By invoking and casting the divine
up as a screen in front of their inability and not having anything to
offer which might help, and so that they might not be clearly revealed
as knowing nothing, they decided that this disease was 'sacred.' And
having selected suitable words, they established their healing methods
with a view towards security for themselves, prescribing purifications and
charms …

In the rest of the treatise, the author goes on to make a number of
observations about human physiology and the nature of the sacred
disease which effectively undermine the position he attributes to all the
charlatans —but what is of interest at this point is his final comment in
the treatise, in which he himself employs the rhetoric of *banausia* against
the healers of another ilk whom he is attacking. In making his emphatic
claim for the intelligibility of the disease and its susceptibility to natural
cures, he states:

> ὅστις δ' ἐπίσταται ἐν ἀνθρώποισι ξηρὸν καὶ ὑγρὸν ποιέειν καὶ θερμὸν καὶ
> ψυχρὸν ὑπὸ διαίτης, οὗτος καὶ ταύτην τὴν νοῦσον ἰῷτο ἄν, εἰ τοὺς καιροὺς
> διαγινώσκοι τῶν συμφερόντων, ἄνευ καθαρμῶν καὶ μαγίης καὶ πάσης τῆς
> τοιαύτης βαναυσίης.   (18.6 Grensemann)

> Whoever understands how to make a person dry and wet and also hot
> and cold by means of a diet, this man also would be able to heal this
> disease, if he understood the opportune times for the helpful materials,
> without purifications and quackery/sorcery and all such *banausia*.

However, even if the author accuses others of practicing *banausia*, this
does not mean that the medical writers in the Hippocratic Corpus shy
away from calling attention to their own status as craftsmen and furthermore as persons who work with their hands: when the author of
the treatise *On Ancient Medicine* defends medicine as a *technê*, he calls
its practitioners *cheirotechnai* and *dêmiourgoi* (ch. 1).[34] To be sure, writers
of Hippocratic treatises are generally more interested in arguing that
medicine is a true *technê* than addressing the question of social status.
Nevertheless, the writers of the Corpus provide good evidence for an
alternative to the dismissive attitudes towards craftsmen held by elitist
writers such as Plato, Aristotle and Xenophon: they very much want
healers to be considered *technitai*, those skilled, knowledgeable workers

---

[34] The author of *On Ancient Medicine* also uses the term *technitês* in chs. 4 and 5 to
describe practitioners of *technai* in general as he argues that healers should be included
in such a classification; for *cheirotechnai* in the Hippocratic Corpus, see also *Affect.* 1 and
45; cf. *cheironax* in *Reg. Acut.* 3 and 11 and *Artic.* 53.

who perform their work with predictable, reliable results. When the medical writers do discuss the role of the healer as it exists in society at large, they express concern about making a good visual impression on both their patients and on the public in general. The treatise *Decorum* exhorts the healer to observe modesty of gesture and dress (and it is interesting that here the writer uses elitist language, urging the healer to be a true nobleman [*kalos kai agathos*, 1]),[35] while in a number of treatises, we learn of the difficulties suffered by the healer faced with an expectant public. So, for example, in *Fractures* 16, the author makes an argument against the use of hollow splints, maintaining that this practice is 'rather lacking in *technê*,' but nonetheless admits that the healer may avoid censure if he uses them—apparently the public find their appearance impressive, and the healer may need to give in to public pressure (πιθανώτερον δὲ τοῖσι δημότῃσίν ἐστι, καὶ τὸν ἰητρὸν ἀναμαρτητότερον εἶναι, ἢν σωλὴν ὑποκέηται· καίτοι ἀτεχνέστερόν γέ ἐστιν).[36]

The medical writers of the Hippocratic Corpus generally proceed with an optimism that is often striking when set in contrast to the expressions of pain and failure found in the poetry of archaic and classical Greece. Furthermore, most of the writers represent themselves as knowledgeable and competent, asserting their ideas about medicine with a dogmatism and confidence that is frequently 'breath-taking.'[37] Although doubts about the effectiveness of a particular treatment are admitted, such deficits are regarded either as manifestations of the harsh realities of nature and human existence or as hurdles that medical science will eventually overcome. So, for example, the author of *The Art* exclaims that medicine, defined as τὸ δὴ πάμπαν ἀπαλλάσσειν τῶν νοσεόντων τοὺς καμάτους καὶ τῶν νοσημάτων τὰς σφοδρότητας ἀμβλύνειν (3.2: 'the complete removal of the sufferings of the sick and the blunting of the excesses of diseases'), is completely capable of achieving this end.[38] The author then argues that in cases where medicine fails to

---

[35] This treatise probably dates to well after the classical period, however (first- to second-century A.D, as stated in Jouanna [1999: 380]), so we must be cautious in using it as evidence for attitudes toward healers in Euripides' day.

[36] For more on the issue of the healer's public appearance and the role of public pressure, see King (1998) 41–45, who emphasizes the concepts of theatricality and deceit that pervade these discussions; see also Jouanna (1999) 75–99.

[37] The adjective used with regard to *The Art* in Lloyd (1987) 116; see also his extensive discussion on the role of dogmatism in the Hippocratic treatises and in Greek science more generally (chapter 3, 'Dogmatism and Uncertainty').

[38] Cf. *Morb. Sacr.* 18.2: οὐδὲν ἄπορόν ἐστιν οὐδ' ἀμήχανον ('there is nothing unintelligible [in any disease] nor untreatable'); *Loc. Hom.* 46.1: ἰητρικὴ δή μοι δοκεῖ ἤδη

heal, it is more likely to be the fault of the patient for refusing to follow
the prescriptions of the *iatros* than the fault of the skilled *iatros* himself
(7). The author does admit that medicine has not yet figured out how to
handle all diseases—internal diseases, he agrees, are still not completely
conquered, but this is because the invisibility of such diseases renders
the task of curing them so difficult (11; even here, some of the blame
lies with the unintelligent patient who is unable to tell the doctor what
he feels). Furthermore, he argues that it is unfair to ask medicine to
cure everything: like any *technê*, medicine has its limits, and there are
some diseases that are—and always will be—beyond the power of the
medical art to cure (8). Healers must not try to exceed their limitations as human beings. Most writers of Hippocratic treatises agree that
some diseases are simply incurable and would concur with the author
of *The Art* when he argues that healers should not even try to cure
patients 'mastered' by disease (8.6) or suffering from diseases deemed
to be incurable (8.4).[39] Furthermore, the medical writers do occasionally express uncertainty, and in some texts, particularly those that are
clinically oriented (and less rhetorically sophisticated), they pause to ask
questions for further research;[40] moreover, they occasionally admit failure. But such admissions, as G.E.R. Lloyd has argued, are not used
to undermine the essential faith the medical writers have in the fundamental soundness of their *technê*; paradoxically, they may serve the
purpose of creating more confidence in scientific principles of the *technê*.
As Lloyd writes:

> '... while detailed accounts of failure in individual cases are confined
> to the more technical works that record actual clinical practice, even
> more theoretical or philosophically oriented treatises occasionally include
> among their otherwise doctrinaire assertions a note to the effect that
> medicine is not certain. With some authors it becomes part of the defini-
> tion of medicine, and of its claim to be the art that it is, that it is inexact.
> The recognition that it cannot do *everything* is sometimes used as a gen-
> uine warning, but it is also sometimes used to bolster claims (and they
> might be extravagant claims) that it *could* do a very great deal.'[41]

ἀνευρῆσθαι ὅλη...βέβηκε γὰρ ἰητρικὴ πᾶσα, καὶ φαίνεται τῶν σοφισμάτων τὰ κάλλιστα ἐν
αὐτῇ συγκείμενα ἐλάχιστα τύχης δεῖσθαι ('for medicine seems to me to have been discovered in its entirety ... for all medicine has progressed, and the most excellent of devices
established in it seem least in need of luck').

[39] See the helpful analysis of the whole issue of incurability in von Staden (1990).
[40] Cf. *Epid.* 2.3.11; 4.25; 6.3.7.
[41] Lloyd (1987) 135.

A distinction is frequently made by writers of the Corpus between the perfection and/or perfectibility of medical *technê* and the deficiencies and faults of its practitioners: when medicine fails, it is usually because it has not been executed properly. Of course, despite this distinction, there remains a tremendous amount of disagreement over correct medical techniques and procedures. But certain commonalities of attitude and definitions of ethical practice exist. First and foremost, healers are to 'help, or at least not to hurt' (ὠφελεῖν ἢ μὴ βλάπτειν) their patients (*Epid.* 1.11) They must observe the patient and look for certain signs; they should examine the patient's urine and feces, substances that exit from the interior of the body and thus provide clues to the unseen inside.[42] A good healer should be able to tell the patient what he or she has already suffered, what he or she is currently experiencing and how the disease will progress in the future. Accurate prognosis is indicative of the healer's knowledge and experience; in some treatises, prognosis seems to be of greater importance to the healer's task, or at least to his reputation, than therapy. The healer should not abuse the trust of his patients (this includes an injunction found in the *Oath* against sexual involvement with a patient). Thus, the good healer tries his best to heal and not to make things worse, is interested foremost in the well-being of his patients, knows how to make prognoses, knows his own limitations, and avoids doing anything which might harm his reputation or the reputation of the profession as a whole.[43]

c. *Heroic measures and the healing art*

During the fifth century, both *technê* itself and the practitioners of *technê* seem to be subject to new scrutiny and evaluation. Hesiod's myth of degeneration (*Works and Days* 109–201) and the optimistic myth of progress presented by fifth-century thinkers such as Protagoras (as Plato

---

[42] For the Presocratic influence on the issue of external signs indicating internal conditions, cf., among others, Anaxagoras DK59 B21a: ὄψις ἀδήλων τὰ φαινόμενα ('apparent things are a vision of unseen ones') and the discussion in Diller (1932).

[43] For more on the theory of *technê* in the Hippocratics, see Roochnik (1996) 42–57, who discusses the ways in which the medical writers must to some extent redefine the meaning of *technê* to accord better with the limitations of their craft: 'The Hippocratic authors acknowledge that their technê is not typical. Their subject matter is alive and, even worse, equipped with an unpredictable and freely operating human will. They realize that as a result their technê cannot achieve, and should not aim for, the sort of clarity, precision, and reliability achieved by other technai' (56).

represents him) and Democritus are set against one another: they not
only compete but intersect.[44] Like Solon, fifth-century authors such as
Euripides emphasize the imperfections of *technê* and the failures of its
practitioners, but they go further in examining the motivations of *technitai* and the problems posed by the existence of *technê* itself. As analyses of the *technê* theme in Greek drama reveal, *technê* may be a sign
of human intelligence, but it can be exploited by the same person for
either good or ill. It may be an essential feature of human civilization,
but that civilization is peopled by humans who may be well-meaning
but incompetent, knowledgeable but mistaken, clever but irresponsible,
or finally skillful but evil. Whereas in the earliest Greek literature, healers do not play a significant role in explorations of the *technê* theme, and
their power to abuse their *technê* is not addressed, the literature of the
fifth century increasingly turns to healers as models for the limitations
and perversions of human intelligence. Healing figures are particularly
useful models with which to explore this topos, I suggest, because of
the peculiar nature of their *technê*. For healers make their living off the
suffering of others, and their *technê* may be acknowledged even by the
healers themselves to be imperfect. Moreover, we begin to see the figure
of the healer used not simply as an example of authoritative behavior
or skilled craftsmanship (and also the negative image of this, with the
failures mentioned by Solon), but also as a participant in more complex metaphors. For example, Agamemnon in Aeschylus likens his role
as a king to that of a healer: he knows how to identify the diseased
elements in society, and to remove them judiciously by cutting or burning (*Agamemnon* 849–850). There are of course several issues which disrupt the king/healer parallel: for one thing, the healer uses these methods to cure others, whereas Agamemnon will do so in order to secure
his own safety and to restore the integrity of his family as rulers. The
parallelism is further undermined by the dramatic context, in which
Agamemnon returns home quite in ignorance of the danger awaiting
him and fails to perceive the signs, and also by Agamemnon's situation
as a returning leader whose position has already been weakened by a
long absence. Indeed, it may be observed that Agamemnon's representation of himself as a healer is inapt. But the Aeschylean metaphor is an
early example of the complex use of healing imagery in the fifth century. Because the object of medical *technê* is the human body itself, there

---

[44] For Protagoras' myth of progress, see Plato, *Prot.* 320c9–322d8; for Democritus,
see especially DK68 B144 and B154. See further discussion in Cole (1967).

is an intense interaction between healers and other humans that is not a necessary part of any other *technê*. The healer claims to have—and must have—the ability to affect immediately and sometimes drastically the life and well being of another individual. As we shall see, this inter-action involves issues of public and private, trust, power, reciprocity and unequal exchange.

Let us now turn to some specific examples of intersections between the tragic view of healers and their *technê* and that represented by the Hippocratic Corpus. I begin with a discussion that focuses on the healer's motivations, but, as will be seen, this quickly brings us into a wide range of associated issues, the most significant of which is that of competence.

If we exclude those few elites who practiced medicine as a kind of benefaction, was there anything beyond family tradition and/or a need to earn a living that motivated a person to become a professional healer in ancient Greece?[45] Clearly, voices in Greek society expressed a need for healers, but was there anything about the profession that actually made it attractive? An *iatromantis* might be divinely inspired to practice his craft, but what of other physicians? As noted above, medical writers were determined to distinguish themselves from less reputable practitioners of the healing arts (as they themselves saw it) and argued long and hard about the nature and status of their pro-fession as a *technê*. Does the *technê* provide some value to the healer as well as the patient? In an important discussion of healers' 'professional ethics,' Ludwig Edelstein argued that the motivation was simple: 'As for the physician's motives in practicing medicine, he was engaged in it in order to make a living.'[46] Thus, according to Edelstein, something like personal morality does not play a role in the practice of ancient Greek medicine. Discussions of ethics in the Hippocratic Corpus focus largely on the construction and maintenance of a good professional reputa-tion: as Heinrich von Staden has recently put it, 'two major motivations shaping the choices, actions and responses of the physician in a variety

---

[45] As happened with other crafts in antiquity, sons (and daughters) often followed their parents into the business; the family of the Asclepiads on Cos is perhaps the best-known example of such a tradition for medical practice. See Burford (1972) 82–88. On how healers organized themselves and how they were educated, see Nutton (1995); for a reconstruction of the career of Hippocrates the Asclepiad *par excellence*, see Jouanna (1999) 1–4, a career that is probably typical in some ways (a family-based business, an itinerant practice) but clearly more illustrious than many.

[46] Edelstein (1956) 324.

of Hippocratic treatises are considerations of *doxa* (that is, of one's professional reputation) and of *technê* (that is, of practising in conformity
with professional expertise).'[47] However, as von Staden goes on to argue
in his persuasive analysis of the Hippocratic *Oath*, at least those healers who swore the oath were indeed committing themselves to integrate
public and private morality in pledging to live both their professional
and personal lives 'in a pure and holy way.' I would like to explore
a passage in another Hippocratic treatise that discusses the nature of
medical *technê*, in order to examine the question of healers' motivations:
in particular, I would like to consider the extent to which healers may
have been inspired by altruism (or, to use Julia Annas' term, 'other-
concern')[48]—or at least tried to represent themselves as inspired by an
unselfish concern for others.

The opening chapter of the Hippocratic treatise *Breaths*, dated by
Jouanna to the last quarter of the fifth century BCE, provides some
intriguing material with which to address this question. This material,
previously quoted in the Introduction, is worth viewing again. The
treatise begins:

> εἰσί τινες τῶν τεχνέων αἳ τοῖσι μὲν κεκτημένοισίν εἰσιν ἐπίπονοι, τοῖσι
> δὲ χρεωμένοισιν ὀνήϊστοι, καὶ τοῖσι μὲν δημότῃσιν ξυνὸν ἀγαθόν, τοῖσι
> δὲ μεταχειριζομένοισί σφας λυπηραί. τῶν δὲ δὴ τοιούτων ἐστὶν τεχνέων
> καὶ ἣν οἱ Ἕλληνες καλέουσιν ἰητρικήν· ὁ μὲν γὰρ ἰητρὸς ὁρεῖ τὰ δεινά,
> θιγγάνει τὰ ἀηδέων, ἐπ᾽ ἀλλοτρίῃσί τε ξυμφορῇσιν ἰδίας καρποῦται λύπας·
> οἱ δὲ νοσέοντες ἀποτρέπονται διὰ τὴν τέχνην τῶν μεγίστων κακῶν, νούσων,
> λύπης, πόνων, θανάτου· πᾶσι γὰρ τούτοισιν ἄντικρυς ἡ ἰητρική.

(1.1–3 Jouanna)

> There are certain *technai* which are grievous for those who practice them,
> but beneficial for those who use them, and while they are a common
> good for the public, they are painful for those who actually do the
> handiwork. Belonging to such a group of *technai* is what the Greeks
> call medical *technê*: for while the healer sees terrible things and touches
> unpleasant ones and reaps his own personal and private pain in the
> sufferings of others, the sick are relieved by means of the *technê* from
> the greatest evils, diseases, grief, toils, death. Opposed to all these things
> is medical *technê*.

The implication that *technê* is valuable and important because it is
directed at both enhancing and preserving human life is certainly not
unusual. Moreover, the author's high praise for medical *technê*, in which

---

[47] Von Staden (1996) 405.
[48] Annas (1993).

he seems to admit little room for its many failures, is, as noted above, typical of discussions of the subject. But the author of *Breaths* introduces two ideas that are not found in other Hippocratic treatises. First, although the idea of the healer as a handworker (emphasized here by the verb *metacheirizesthai*) is a common one, as we have seen, the author of *Breaths* emphasizes the personal pain and suffering of the healer in contrast to the achievement of the common good. As discussed earlier in the Introduction, suffering from the suffering of others is a common topos in the fifth century.[49] But the medical writers usually observe suffering with an objective rather than a subjective gaze; the role of the healer is to impress the patient with his competence and instill confidence by appearing sensible and unperturbed. Although they argue that their role is an important one, it is nonetheless acknowledged to be ancillary: the main struggle takes place between the patient and the disease. So, for example, in the triangular relationship proposed by the author of *Epidemics* 1, the healer takes on the role of assistant to the *technê*, while it is the patient who does the actual fighting of the disease, with the healer's help: ἡ τέχνη διὰ τριῶν, τὸ νούσημα, ὁ νοσέων, καὶ ὁ ἰητρός· ὁ ἰητρός, ὑπηρέτης τῆς τέχνης· ὑπεναντιοῦσθαι τῷ νουσήματι τὸν νοσεῦντα μετὰ τοῦ ἰητροῦ χρή. (11: 'The *technê* consists of three factors: the disease, the patient, and the healer: the healer is the servant of the *technê*: it is necessary that the patient oppose the disease with the help of the healer').[50] By contrast, the author of *Breaths* gives the healer a starring role in the struggle: he assigns pain to the healer and relief to the patient.[51]

As to the second point, the writer calls attention to the manual activity of the healer in a more negative way than his fellow writers, when he points out that the healer must touch disagreeable things (presumably the sweat, urine, feces, and other bodily substances that we often hear discussed in the rest of the Corpus). It should be observed how rarely the authors of the Corpus mention personal feelings of distaste in their

---

[49] Cf., as noted in the Introduction, passages from Gorgias (DK82 B11[9]) and the *Dissoi Logoi* (DK90 1 [3]).

[50] For a study that examines the different sides of this 'triangular' relationship as it operated in the Roman period, see Gourevitch (1984).

[51] *Breath's* author emphasizes not only the tactile elements of his art, but also the visual ones, as though he were in the spectacle of a tragedy. The healer acts both as a spectator, seeing terrible things (ὁρεῖ τὰ δεινά), and as a participant in the sufferings (ξυμφοραί) of his patients. The author claims moreover that the skill of the healer cures great evils which he defines as 'νοῦσαι, λύπη, πόνοι, θάνατος,' evils that are the very stuff of tragedy. On this point, see also Jouanna (1987) 109.

observations of patients. They do discuss patients' feelings of shame and disgrace, as for example in the description of the epileptic sufferer in *On the Sacred Disease*, who hides his face in shame (12). As noted above, they also discuss proper comportment for themselves and urge healers both to appear graceful and authoritative in person and to make their attentions to the patient, whether in positioning the body or putting on a bandage, attractive in appearance. But for persons so attuned to the importance of beauty in Greek culture, the authors of the Corpus maintain a remarkably clinical and impersonal attitude towards what our author suggests are indeed unpleasant things to deal with. Thus, it is striking that at the same time the author of *Breaths* places the healer onto the noble plane of generous service to the community, he reminds us of what exactly it is that healers may have to do in the course of such service.

What, in fact, is the goal of this argument? Why does the author judge it to be appealing or important that healers suffer and gain nothing from their exertions on behalf of others except for personal pain? Furthermore, why the stress on the unpleasant experiences necessitated by the physical interaction with patients? The author seems to be urging us to admire the healer for engaging in painful and even repellent activities. I am making no radical claim when I say that arguments based on pure altruism (certainly in its Kantian form) are rare in archaic and classical Greece, at least before Aristotle; it is normally assumed that even when performing beneficial tasks for others, the 'good-deed doer' will win something for himself, whether that be glory, booty, power or exemption from certain taxes.[52] The idea of reciprocity, whether immediate and 'balanced' or expected in the long run and so 'generalized,' remains a powerful force in motivating Greek behavior.[53] So in Homer, where the Greeks continued to look for their models of appropriate behavior even when their social structures had changed

---

[52] On the history of 'other-concern,' see Annas (1993) especially part 3, who argues that the history of Greek ethical thought shows a change in the evaluation of actions done in the interests of others, a change that begins with Aristotle, whose works set certain ethical standards to which later thinkers had to respond. On altruism/ 'other-concern' in heroic epic, see discussion in Zanker (1994) 131–154, with further discussion in Zanker (1998); he argues that a form of altruism, which he calls magnanimity ('disinterested generosity') is represented by the actions of Achilles at the end of the *Iliad*. For arguments against understanding such activity as a form of altruism, see the essays of Gill and Postlethwaite in Gill, Postlethwaite and Seaford (1998).

[53] For the definitions and analyses of the terms 'balanced' and 'generalized' reciprocity, see Donlan (1981–1982).

enormously, we find support for acting with pity and with generosity, but not much for suffering on behalf of others with no expectation of benefit in return: for example, at *Iliad* 20.297–298, Poseidon criticizes Aeneas for fighting with Achilles, saying: ἀλλὰ τί ἢ νῦν οὗτος ἀναίτιος ἄλγεα πάσχει /μὰψ ἕνεκ' ἀλλοτρίων ἀχέων ... ('But why now does this man, who is blameless, suffer pains / for no reason, for the sake of the unhappiness of others ...?'). On the other hand, as evidence for Greek understanding of and sympathy for altruistic behavior, Zanker points to Aristotle's discussions of mothers who sacrifice themselves on behalf of their children (*Nichomachean Ethics* 1159a28–33) and his analysis of *charis* in *Rhetoric* 1381b35–37 as an unadvertised and unsolicited favor for a friend, and later on his definition of *charis* 'as the emotion of benevolence or kindliness displayed when one renders a favor to fulfill a real need, without the expectation of a return favor, and without any self-interest on the part of the donor (1385a17–19).'[54] Even in Aristotle, though, as Gill argues, we are dealing with actions performed not on behalf of *anyone*, but rather in the context of social 'solidarity'—that is, in the context of the maintenance or establishment of communal friendships or in the context of familial obligations and needs.[55] To interpret the appeal of the statement in *Breaths* to a fifth-century audience, it will be useful to examine some other contexts in which the ideas put forward by the author appear. Such a discussion will bring us more fully into the literature of the classical period and indeed into the heart of our analysis proper. The writer's statement, I argue, has connotations that are worked out in positive and negative directions in two tragedies, Aeschylus' *Prometheus Bound* and Euripides' *Hippolytus*. In the analysis that follows, I will first examine *Prometheus Bound*, whose protagonist, the culture-bringer Prometheus, I suggest, serves as a model for the heroic *iatros* described by the author of *Breaths* and then proceed to a discussion of the negative treatment of the healing role that occurs in Euripides' *Hippolytus*.

[54] Zanker (1994) 132–133.
[55] Gill (1998); on Aristotle, see 317–323. For a critique of Gill and a further exploration of the concept of altruism in antiquity, see Konstan (2000).

CHAPTER TWO

HEALERS IN GREEK TRAGEDY

a. Prometheus Bound: *The healer as philanthropist*

In his opening statement, the author of *Breaths* brings together the elite
ideology of bestowing benefits on the community despite some personal
cost and the somewhat contrary belief in the extraordinary power and
importance of *technê*; at the same time, he refers to the unpleasant tasks
undertaken by medical practitioners. In so doing, it seems to me, he
is setting up a particular model of good behavior, a model that goes
beyond the kind of generosity that is afforded by the elite. It is not a
model that aims merely for the reward of honor and privilege (*timê*), but
rather sets before itself the larger and more difficult task of improving
human culture; not, then, of maintaining society in good stead, of
sustaining order and traditional values, but in fact of making society
better. This model of behavior goes beyond the goals of most Homeric
heroes, even the craftsman Odysseus; instead it looks, as I have said, to
the figure of the culture bringer that can be seen most clearly in the
Prometheus Bound, which I would now like to examine briefly.

The play opens with Prometheus being chained to the rock, pun-
ished by Zeus because he gave fire to mortals. In Hesiod's version of
the tale, Prometheus restores fire to humankind after Zeus has deprived
them of it (*Works and Days* 42–52). Hesiod also describes a rather different aftermath: the gift of fire results ultimately in the great suffering
of mortals since Zeus devises the punishment of Pandora and her box,
whence spring thousands of ills for humankind.[1] In *Prometheus Bound,*

---

[1] On the differences between the Hesiodic and Aeschylean accounts of the Prometheus myth, see Conacher (1980) 3–15, who states as the fundamental distinction
between the two, 'the Hesiodic Prometheus ... is presented (however "artificially") as
the indirect cause of all man's woes; the Aeschylean Prometheus, on the other hand, ...
is presented as the saviour of mankind, without whom man would have ceased to exist
and with whose help he progresses from mere subsistence to a state of civilization' (13).
Saïd (1985: 103) generally agrees with the contrast worked out by Conacher, but she
goes on to demonstrate that the civilizing arts of Prometheus are not depicted in such a

however, it seems at least at the start of the play that only Prometheus
will suffer for his actions. Moreover, in contrast to the degeneration of
mortal life that ensues after the gift of fire in Hesiod, *Prometheus Bound*
tells a story of human progress made possible by the compassion and
generosity of Prometheus.[2] Indeed, fire is just the first of the many gifts
to mortals that Prometheus and the chorus will tell us about in the play.
Zeus in this play is represented as a cruel tyrant interested only in his
own power, whereas Prometheus has taken pity on mortals, even going
so far as to side with them against the gods when the gods, led by Zeus,
attempted to destroy them entirely. Cratus, who enters with Hephaes-
tus at the start of the play to perform the act of binding Prometheus,
states that it is being done so that Prometheus will learn to cherish the
tyranny of Zeus and cease from his human-loving manner, his *philanthrôpos tropos*.[3]

---

positive light in Aeschylus; see more on this below. For a discussion that focuses on the
structural similarities of the two versions, see Detienne and Vernant (1978) 133–174.

  [2] To be sure, that progress towards civilization is not complete: as a number of
studies have shown, human society in *PV* still awaits the *dikê* and *aidôs* and the *politikê
technê* that are necessary elements in the concept of civilization that is rehearsed in
ancient accounts of the myth of progress (especially as told in Plato's *Protagoras*). The
cleft between knowledge (Prometheus) and power (Zeus) illustrated in *PV* needs to be
resolved in order to achieve human civilization. On the state of human knowledge in
the play and the gaps that exist in the gifts given by Prometheus, see Saïd (1985) 138–
154 and 342–343, who also notes the emphasis placed on the utter passivity of humans
in this account. Other stories of human progress place greater emphasis on nature,
necessity and human inventiveness in devising technological advances; see Cole (1967)
and Dodds (1973).

  [3] The word *philanthrôpos* and its compounds occur rarely in extant Greek literature
up through the fifth century, appearing first here in *PV*. Plato has Socrates use the word
in *Euthyphro* 3d7, a passage that emphasizes the suggestions of self-denial and lack of
ordinary concern for self-interest: Socrates jokes that because of his *philanthrôpia*, he is
open to conversing with anyone, not only without expecting payment, but also perhaps
even willing to pay others for their company. Plato also uses the word in association
with healing imagery at *Symposium* 189d1–3, where Aristophanes describes Eros: ἔστι γὰρ
θεῶν φιλανθρωπότατος, ἐπίκουρός τε ὢν τῶν ἀνθρώπων καὶ ἰατρὸς τούτων ὧν ἰαθέντων
μεγίστη εὐδαιμονία ἂν τῷ ἀνθρωπείῳ γένει εἴη ('He is the most human loving of gods,
being both a helper of humankind and a healer of those things the cure of which is
the greatest blessing for the human race.'). Use of the word flourishes in the orators
of the fourth century, where it is used in a complimentary sense to describe behavior
that is 'kind' or 'humane': it connotes generosity of spirit (cf., e.g., Arist. *EN* 1155a20;
Dem. *In Mid.* 48–49). The word also occurs in the opening section of one of the later
treatises of the Hippocratic Corpus, *Physician* (late fourth-century), to describe how the
iatros should act towards his patients, while the treatise *Precepts* explains that *philanthrôpia*
is an essential component of *philotechnia* (6). On *philanthrôpia* and medicine, see Temkin
(1991) 23–35.

Prometheus, as his name suggests, also has the gift of prophecy; as the play progresses, we learn that he knows of a great threat to Zeus' power, but he refuses to tell it. Both Zeus, the tyrant, and Prometheus, the human-lover, are entrenched in their positions, with Prometheus both refusing to submit to Zeus' authority and asserting the appropriateness of his actions for all concerned, and Zeus refusing to soften his harsh stance in any way. Prometheus, in one of many uses of disease imagery in the play,[4] characterizes Zeus' hateful attitude towards him as a *nosêma*, a disease that is typical of tyranny (224–225). When the character Oceanus urges Prometheus to try softer methods, such as persuading words, to heal Zeus' sick anger, Prometheus answers that he will heal Zeus' disease when the time is right:

> Ὠκέανος. οὔκουν, Προμηθεῦ, τοῦτο γιγνώσκεις, ὅτι
> ὀργῆς νοσούσης εἰσὶν ἰατροὶ λόγοι;
> Προμηθεύς. ἐάν τις ἐν καιρῷ γε μαλθάσσῃ κέαρ
> καὶ μὴ σφριγῶντα θυμὸν ἰσχναίνῃ βίᾳ.　　　　　(377–380)

> Okeanos. Do you not therefore recognize this fact, Prometheus, that
> words are the healers of a sick anger?
> Prometheus. If one softens the heart at the right moment at any rate
> and does not try to reduce with violence a spirit that is swelling up.

The members of the chorus, largely sympathetic to Prometheus, nevertheless seem to shake their heads in wonder over his determination to stick by his position and over his boldness in helping mortals in the past. For his part, Prometheus bemoans the irony that while he gave many *technai* to mortals so that they might overcome difficulties, he himself can find no *sophisma*, no clever plan (470), to extract himself from the situation. In response to such remarks, the chorus compares him to a poor doctor who cannot heal himself:

> κακὸς δ' ἰατρὸς ὥς τις ἐς νόσον
> πεσὼν ἀθυμεῖς, καὶ σεαυτὸν οὐκ ἔχεις
> εὑρεῖν ὁποίοις φαρμάκοις ἰάσιμος.　　　　　(473–475)

> Like some bad healer falling sick
> you are dispirited and you are not able
> to discover by what drugs you yourself are curable.

---

[4] The medical imagery in the play is striking and has been thoroughly discussed by Dumortier (1935). See also the sensible discussion in Saïd (1985) 168–186, who uses the work of Dumortier with appropriate caution (see, e.g., 169; 172; 173 n. 121), and see the many Hippocratic parallels noted by Guardasole (2000) 40–55 and 160–176.

Prometheus acknowledges this while pointing out the further irony that it was he who instructed human beings in the art of medicine. The members of the chorus are admiring of his philanthropic activities, yet they also emphasize the inability of puny mortals to help Prometheus in return for these benefits and wonder what he has gained from all this: as they state in a choral ode,

φέρ' ὅπως χάρις ἀ χάρις, ὦ φίλος,
εἰπέ, ποῦ τις ἀλκά;
τίς ἐφαμερίων ἄρηξις;   (545–547)

Come now, friend, say how the favor (that you did) is a favor,
where is some aid (for you)?
What help from mortals is there (for you)?

Despite the fact that he appears to reap no personal gain from helping others with their sufferings, Prometheus continues his compassionate ways in the scene with the pregnant and distraught Io who appears late in the play; although he cannot assuage her physical pain, he provides comfort by predicting what will happen to her.[5] At the end of the play, however, we are no closer to resolving the situation between Prometheus and Zeus; indeed, the situation escalates and greater violence threatens. It seems likely that in the later plays of the trilogy, a reconciliation took place and Zeus introduced justice and law into human society, gifts which Prometheus, the technician, did not have the capacity to give them.[6]

As this brief sketch has shown, the play provides a model for self-sacrificing behavior on a grand scale in the character of Prometheus. Prometheus, the chorus maintains, gave his gifts of various *technai* to mortals out of compassion, without hope of or interest in gain, without expectation of favors in return, and at the cost of intense personal

---

[5] Saïd (1985: 179–186) argues that the failure of *technê* to cure Io (and to help Prometheus) indicates the impotence of *technê* in the absence of power, especially divine power. While I agree that the play speaks to the limitations of *technê* (and certainly as concerns the character of Prometheus himself), the importance placed by Hippocratic healers on prognosis should not be overlooked; indeed, when one considers the inability of healers in antiquity to heal any number of serious diseases, it is not surprising that they should place special emphasis on their powers of prediction as an essential element of their *technê*. Saïd herself discusses the role of prognosis in medical *technê*, but argues that the role of prognosis in the play, although expressed frequently in the medical language, is closer to the category of mantic *technê* (192–195). The power of foreknowledge is emphasized in the play, but this was also seen by Hippocratics as part of medical *technê*.

[6] For this interpretation and its history, see Conacher (1980) 92–97.

suffering. As a Titan, he has greater status than mere mortals, so perhaps we might say that his actions are in accord with the expectations of members of the elite class. Now of course we can also interpret Prometheus' actions as self-interested in that they further his own ends in a great power struggle with Zeus. And surely that is part of the story, too. At the same time, however, we see the characters around him surprised that he does not have greater regard for his own personal interests. They interpret his actions as having no personal motive. In a play where the divisions between power and knowledge, compassion and violence, submission and resistance are all represented in extremes, the motivations of Prometheus in helping humans are likewise revealed as extraordinary.[7] His *technai* fail to help him, but they do help others. His acts of compassion, his use of *technai*, are greater than what one could expect from someone with a normal scale of values; they provoke not only wonder, but also admiration—indeed, the chorus of Oceanids, who wonder at his behavior, are nonetheless inspired at the end of the play to support his position even if it means their own destruction (1063–1070). I suggest that the author of *Breaths* is working from a similar perspective as he opens his treatise: he is laying claim to a particular form of heroic status, the status of culture-bringer.

The direct involvement of medical *technê* in the development of civilization is not, of course, unique among Hippocratic authors to the author of *Breaths*: section 3 of the treatise *On Ancient Medicine* contains an extended discussion of medicine's role in human progress. In an analysis of the evolutionary theory advanced in the treatise, Jackie Pigeaud has suggested that the author of *On Ancient Medicine* believes that disease arose in the world in order to force human society to evolve, that the presence of disease acted as a catalyst for the development of human social institutions; thus, disease has a positive function as an instigator of human culture and human progress, a *pathos* (suffering) that lead to

---

[7] Saïd (1985) contrasts the utter lack of pity and concern shown by Zeus towards mortals in *PV* with the attitudes of divinities in the *Iliad* and *Odyssey* (246–258). She notes that even given that gods in Homer show interest in and compassion for human beings, such emotions are most often directed at an individual or a city—but not towards the entire human race (or, to use Gill's expression, '*anyone*'), and she emphasizes the unusual attitude of Prometheus, especially since the absence of reciprocity is so marked: 'L'attitude de Prométhée est d'autant plus étonnante que sa φιλότης et son εὔνοια pour les mortels n'ont, dans le cadre de la tragédie, aucune justification, car rien n'indique qu'il ait créé les hommes ou qu'il ait eu à réparer un tort qu'il leur aurait causé' (258).

mathos (learning).[8] The author of *Breaths*, by contrast, looks to a different model, where it is the healers who are teachers, rather than the disease. The author of the treatise *Breaths* attempts to bridge the gap between elite and popular notions of *technê*. He combines arguments that will appeal to the ideologies of status prevalent in classical Greece with a particular claim not only for the value of *technê* itself but also for the importance of its practitioners.

This discussion does not presuppose that all healers were motivated by self-sacrifice. Furthermore, self-sacrifice must not be confused with altruism, which, in Gill's definition, extends itself towards *anyone*. However, remarks in other treatises lend themselves to the notion that some form of altruism was at least ideally a part of Greek medical ethics: thus, the treatise *Precepts* contains an injunction to heal people with or without monetary compensation (6), and the *Oath* directs the good behavior of those who swear it towards just about '*anyone*,' as von Staden has noted in his analysis:

> Its promises extend though three generations of human healers (2.i–v) to all persons, regardless of gender and social or civic status (7.ii). They extend to all of the ill without qualification (3.i, 7.i). Moreover, the *Oath* applies not only to all therapeutic relations with other humans but also to all non-therapeutic interactions (8.i). It covers all human dwellings that the oath-taker might ever enter (7.i), regardless of whom he might encounter in them. Furthermore, the *Oath* extends over all things that its reciter 'might see or hear' (8.i)—a disjunctive formal that expresses comprehensiveness—and, in his relations with others, the oath-taker undertakes to be 'far from *all* voluntary, destructive injustice.'[9]

Moreover, the words of *Breaths*' author do seem to find an historical analogue in a passage from Thucydides, a passage which at the same time reveals the limits of medical *technai* in classical Greece. This passage is taken from the beginning of Thucydides' description of the plague at Athens:

---

[8] Pigeaud (1990). Hence, the author of *On Ancient Medicine* seems to suggest that a kind of combination of the *pathei mathos* ('learning through suffering') idea found in tragedy (the phrase occurs perhaps most memorably at *Agamemnon* 177) and the theory of progress advanced by Protagoras. Pigeaud also suggests that the views expressed in *On Ancient Medicine* provide a contrast to other texts of the Corpus: thus, for example, the author of *On the Sacred Disease* denies any purpose for disease at all. And, while indicating that humans can bring disease upon themselves through improper behavior, the other treatises of the Corpus do not suggest that disease arose in the world in order to teach humans responsibility or respect for the gods and human law.

[9] Von Staden (1996) 435. The numbers in the quoted passage refer to von Staden's own division of the phrases of the text of the *Oath*.

οὔτε γὰρ ἰατροὶ ἤρκουν τὸ πρῶτον θεραπεύοντες ἀγνοίᾳ (ἀλλ' αὐτοὶ μάλιστα ἔθνῃσκον ὅσῳ καὶ μάλιστα προσῇσαν), οὔτε ἄλλη ἀνθρωπεία τέχνη
οὐδεμία, ὅσα τε πρὸς ἱεροῖς ἱκετεῦσαν ἢ μαντείοις καὶ τοῖς τοιούτοις ἐχρή-
σαντο πάντα ἀνωφελῆ ἦν. τελευτῶντές τε αὐτῶν ἀπέστησαν ὑπὸ τοῦ κακοῦ
νικώμενοι.   (2.47.4)

For the healers were not up to the task, since they were treating the
disease for the first time in ignorance (but they themselves died especially
to the extent that they especially came into contact [with the disease]),
nor was any other human *technê* of use: however much people prayed
at shrines or made use of divinations and such things, everything was
unhelpful. In the end, overwhelmed by the catastrophe, they stopped
fighting against it.

Here we see compassion linked paradoxically with both *technê* and
agnoia, ignorance. The contrast with the optimism of the Hippocratic
author is striking: he maintains that the doctors in their compassion
will suffer private pains from the suffering of others, but nevertheless
he asserts the power of the *technê* itself to free the patient from disease,
suffering, toil, and death itself. But as Thucydides' horrifying description of the plague reveals, the doctors were all too often powerless
against the forces of disease and were all the more affected by the disease because of their efforts. Despite the many warnings found in the
Hippocratic Corpus about avoiding intervention in desperate cases, it
is clear that the doctors tried their best in the case of the plague. Scholars have shown that Thucydides was strongly influenced by rationalist
medical thinking, but the few statements that he actually makes about
doctors are skeptical with regard to their abilities.[10] Nevertheless, in the
description of the plague, Thucydides portrays the doctors as members
of a very small group of people who stood by their sense of honor and
continued to practice appropriate human *nomoi*. Surely if we are to seek
for examples of both heroism and 'other-concern' in classical Greek
antiquity, we do find one such example here.

b. *Euripides'* Hippolytus: *The charlatan in action*

The opening words of *Breaths* make use of a topos which, while not
unique in the literature of the Greek classical period, is nevertheless
somewhat unusual. Jouanna cites Aristophanes *Wealth* 706 in support of

---

[10] On Thucydides' estimation of healers, see Herter (1966). There is copious literature on Thucydides and medicine: see especially Rechenauer (1991).

the notion that the healer's task is a disagreeable one and also points to the words of the Nurse at *Hippolytus* 186–188, a correspondence noted by Wilamowitz in his commentary on the play: κρεῖσσον δὲ νοσεῖν ἢ θεραπεύειν·/ τό μέν ἐστιν ἁπλοῦν, τῷ δὲ συνάπτει/ λύπη τε φρενῶν χερσίν τε πόνος ('it is better to be sick than to provide care for the sick: for the former is a single issue, but in the latter case, pain of the mind and labor with the hands combine'). Like the author of *Breaths*, the Nurse emphasizes not only the mental suffering of the healer, but also the issue of manual labor. However, Euripides also shows us how such a topos can be manipulated and placed into a particularly negative context. We should notice first that the Nurse's argument is slightly different than that of *Breaths*' author and second from whose lips the argument stems. The Nurse maintains that it is *better* to be sick than to be a care-giver, since sickness is a singular issue whereas the care-giver experiences the two-fold suffering of mental anguish and physical toil. Scholars analyzing the Nurse's language have shown its heavy use of sophistic rhetoric; at the same time, they have stressed the importance of her lower class status for the correct understanding of her role.[11] The model of medicine practiced by the Nurse is based on a single goal, the preservation of the patient's life: as she says when Phaidra protests against her therapeutic suggestions, νῦν δ' ἀγὼν μέγας, / σῶσαι βίον σόν, κοὺκ ἐπίφθονον τόδε (496–497: 'now we are engaged in a great struggle—to save your life, and this is not despicable'). Like the healer in *Breaths*, the Nurse aims to free her patient from death, but her method is purely pragmatic and devoid of moral consideration, or rather, her sense of proper behavior differs emphatically from not only from standard Greek norms of proper behavior (after all, her advice is to urge her charge to commit adultery), but also from the code of ethics promulgated by the healers whose views are represented in the Hippocratic Corpus. According to that code of practice, as mentioned above, a healer is 'to be useful, or at least to do no harm' (ὠφελεεῖν ἢ μὴ βλάπτειν, *Epid.* 1.11).[12] Furthermore, the healer should realize the

---

[11] See McClure (1999) 135–141.

[12] The famous language of the Hippocratic *Oath* would also be useful to cite here: not only does it contain the injunction 'not to harm,' but also instructs the healer about the importance of doctor-patient confidentiality, surely violated by the Nurse. However, because the date of the *Oath* is much disputed (cf. Jouanna [1999] 401) we must be cautious not to make too much of any parallels between it and tragedy: it is certainly possible that such confidentiality was a common and long-standing practice among healers, but we cannot know for certain.

limitations of his *technê* and refrain from intervening when the disease is beyond the power of medicine to heal.[13] While numerous cultural referents no doubt inform Euripides' portrait of the Nurse, I suggest that Euripides has based this character not only on the model of a sophist but also on the model of a healer, a healer who claims to suffer in tending her patient, but fails to free her patient from any pain or disease at all; in fact, her actions precipitate her patient's death through suicide. Indeed, the *Hippolytus*, among its many virtues, gives us a fairly well-developed sketch of an incompetent healer, who unwittingly uses the rhetoric found in *Breaths* and other treatises of the Hippocratic Corpus for all the wrong purposes.[14]

The *Hippolytus*, at least in the first half of the play, is replete with words and images common also to the language of medical texts. It is a play in which language is at once as problematic and as effective as action, and the medical language used in the play is no exception. The word *nosos* is a case in point: as Barrett comments,[15] *nosos* refers sometimes to Phaedra's self-induced sickness (the disease which she brings upon herself in her attempt to die) and sometimes to her love for Hippolytus (love-sickness). What Barrett does not say is that the word is in fact used in distinctive ways by the different speakers. Phaedra, who uses the word three times, twice uses it to denote her love for Hippolytus (394, 405) and once in the more generalized sense of 'suffering' (730—this only after her love has been exposed to Hippolytus himself). The Nurse, however, always uses the word *nosos* to refer to Phaedra's sickness or to sickness in general. This ambiguity is significant for our understanding of Phaedra's reaction to the Nurse's offer of *pharmaka*. Phaedra believes—or at least hopes—that the Nurse intends to cure her of her love; the Nurse, however, intends to cure her of her disease. Curing the sickness brought on by love is perhaps in the realm of possibilities for a healer; curing love itself is far more difficult. In this play, neither disease is overcome by *pharmaka*; instead, only death provides any kind of remedy.

The Nurse is established in her first speech as someone familiar with the contemporary rhetoric of the medical profession, although

---

[13] See, e.g., *Fract.* 36, *Ars* 3, 8, *Prog.* 1 and discussion in von Staden (1990).

[14] As we shall see in analyses of other Euripidean plays, the Nurse is not the only incompetent healer represented in Euripidean drama; nonetheless, this Euripidean character-type is most fully developed in *Hippolytus*.

[15] Commentary *ad* 476–477.

her language is more pessimistic and less precise than that used in the Hippocratic Corpus. She expresses doubts about the possibility of remedy: as she maintains at 189–190, the whole of human life is painful (*odynêros*) and there is no ceasing from labors/pains (*ponoi*). The term *ponos* with its broad semantic range is certainly not confined to medical discourse; however, it is a standard term in the Hippocratic Corpus for dull, recurring or chronic pain. By contrast, the noun *odynê* is a 'sharp, shooting pain.'[16] Rarely occurring in tragedy, which prefers less concrete or prosaic words for pain such as *algos*, it is the most common word for pain in the Hippocratic Corpus. In her analysis of these two terms, King suggests that *ponos*, which according to Hesiod is an integral part of life in the Age of Iron, refers to acceptable levels of pain, pain for which 'it may be considered culturally inappropriate to offer pain relief'; *odynê*, by contrast, is pain beyond what is expected and thus admits of treatment.[17] The Nurse's speech combines both forms of pain as she speaks of the misery of human existence. Even if both *ponos* and *odynêros* are used metaphorically elsewhere in tragedy, it is likely that the Nurse is using them in a physical sense here, for the Nurse's primary concern—in contrast to Phaedra's anguished moral reflections—turns out to be the preservation of physical well-being. Even though her arguments often point to contemporary discussions among the *sophoi* and their discussions of ethical matters, her focus is on pure bodily existence. Although initially alarmed by Phaedra's disclosure that she loves Hippolytus, the Nurse soon finds plenty of arguments to counter her patient's moral scruples (which she dismisses with the question, τί σεμνομυθεῖς;, 490: 'why do you preach?'); such seemingly illicit love must in fact be natural and appropriate, she asserts, since it is practiced by divinities. For the Nurse, life itself, painful as it may be, is the essential issue, not how to live it; moral principles are well and good when one is healthy or at ease, but Phaedra is engaged in a struggle for

---

[16] Rey (1995) 21. The adjective form *odynêros* is rare and usually metaphorical in literary texts: it describes old age at Mimnermus 1.5–6 and poverty at 2.12; elsewhere it is used once of wealth (Eur. *Phoen.* 566) and once of ignorance (Theognis *Elegies* 1.896). The adjective also occurs infrequently in the Hippocratic Corpus: it describes ear pain at *Artic.* 40 and *Coac.* 195 (in adverbial form). It becomes much more common in later medical authors such as Galen. Its usage in connection with *ponos* in this passage may emphasize a physical rather than a metaphorical pain.

[17] King (1998) 125; on ancient attitudes towards pain, see King (1989) and (1998) 117–131. But see also the critique of King's argument on the vocabulary of pain in Horden (1999).

her life. Her argument may perhaps have struck a chord in some members of the audience in 428 BCE, who had just suffered through the plague: for the Athenians at this time, the basic preservation of life in the face of disease was never of more central importance. Nevertheless, the social crisis which the plague precipitated made it clear, at least to Thucydides, the absolute necessity of moral principles which regulated self and society and defined a life as worthwhile.[18] Phaedra, indeed, resists the theory that the behavior of the gods countenances transgression against mortal *nomoi*. Moreover, she defines her love as a kind of *miasma* in her *phrên* (a 'pollution' in her 'emotional center,' 317);[19] believing that she cannot be cleansed, she has condemned herself to death. Phaedra's ethics, which center on her concern for her good name and reputation for *aidôs* (shame and respect),[20] clash with the Nurse's belief in the value of life, no matter how it is lived.

Until the Nurse urges Phaedra to give in to love, we might be tempted to think of her as a stubborn and fussy old woman, solicitous of her mistress' welfare and basically innocuous. But Euripides in fact provides us with some hints that the Nurse is in fact something more—and something more problematic. The Nurse is prone to giving advice, much of which corresponds to advice found in treatises of the Hippocratic Corpus. Thus, she admonishes her patient not to move around so much, for the disease will be easier to withstand if she lies quietly (203–206).[21] Later, as she obeys Phaedra's wish to have her head covered, the Nurse comments:

---

[18] Thucydides describes the breakdown of standards of correct behavior during the plague (such as the abuse of burial practices reported at 2.52.3–4) together with the manipulation of language; while he does not directly state that moral principles and a set of standards for behavior are absolutely necessary for the flourishing of a society, he certainly implies this.

[19] For the meaning(s) of *phrên* in Greek literature, see Padel (1992) 20–23, who emphasizes that *phrenes* are also organs of thought and knowledge—but always with an emotional element. For a medical discussion in antiquity that gives insight into common perceptions of the *phrên*, see *On the Sacred Disease* 17, where the author attacks those who believe people think with their *phrên*, rather than with their brain.

[20] There is a huge literature on Phaedra's moral reflections—and on her culpability— in this play: for a useful discussion of her moral stance with an emphasis both on the meaning of *aidôs* and on the role of the Nurse in defining appropriate behavior in the play, see Cairns (1993) 314–340.

[21] For the advice to abstain from movement in illness using the word ἡσυχία or variants of the same stem, see, for example, *Intern.* 1, 2, 3, 6, 8, 10, 12, 15, 17; *Nat. Mul.* 44; *Morb. Mul.* 2.118, 149.

πολλὰ διδάσκει μ' ὁ πολὺς βίοτος·
χρῆν γὰρ μετρίας εἰς ἀλλήλους
φιλίας θνητοὺς ἀνακίρνασθαι
καὶ μὴ πρὸς ἄκρον μυελὸν ψυχῆς,
εὔλυτα δ' εἶναι στέργηθρα φρενῶν
ἀπό τ' ὤσασθαι καὶ ξυντεῖναι·   (252–257)

> My long life teaches me many things: for it would be better that mortals
> mix in moderate friendships with one another and not to the deep
> marrow of the soul, but bonds of emotion should be easy to dissolve,
> both to push apart and to bind together.

Key words here are *metria philia* and *anakirnasthai*: the Nurse is a believer
in the balanced mixture school of health.[22] The word *eulyta*, too, especially in combination with ἀπό τ' ὤσασθαι καὶ ξυντεῖναι, reveals the
Nurse's ability to manipulate medical discourse: she speaks of love as
though it were a material substance which can be 'easily dissolved' and
'pushed out' if it is not too deeply embedded in the 'marrow of the soul'
(πρὸς ἄκρον μυελὸν ψυχῆς).[23] She goes on to reiterate in different words
her earlier statement that it is more difficult to be doctor than patient,
asserting now that the doctor figure suffers doubly in suffering for him
or herself as well as for the patient (258–260).

---

[22] This is a common tenet of the Hippocratic Corpus, although it is found first in the
words of the Presocratic Alcmaeon of Croton (DK24 B4), on which see more below in
Part II (p. 158); cf., e.g., *Reg.* 1.3–8. Many rationalist thinkers found their explanation for
the causes of disease in a theory of essential elements—that is to say, they argued that
the human body is at root comprised of some number of basic elements, usually two or
four, which are mixed together in different ways to form the body as a whole. Not every
author uses the same group of elements in his theory, but the theories almost always
choose from the same list: either a set of qualities, very often wet, cold, warm, dry,
bitter, sweet, and salty, or a combination of the so-called humors—water, blood, yellow
bile, black bile, and phlegm. The balance or harmony of these elements brings health,
the predominance of a single element results in illness. The healthiest individuals are
those whose bodies have the most balanced blend of different elements, yet most people
tend to have constitutions slightly dominated by one of them. The healer intervenes
therefore either preventatively to maintain balance or *ex post facto* to restore it.
[23] *Eulytos* in particular is very much a prosaic word, frequently found in the Hippocratic Corpus and other medical texts, but occurring only here in poetic texts of the
archaic and classical periods. On *myelos* in the Corpus and in fifth-century tragedy, see
Guardasole (2000) 91–98.
  It is important to emphasize that the Nurse does not at this point know that Phaedra
is in love with Hippolytus. She first uses the term *philia*, which denotes a non-erotic
form of love, and then *stergêthra phrenôn*, which refer to desires and passions generally
and are not confined to erotic love. However, these are desires of the *phrên* and not of
the *nous*; to that extent, they need have no rational basis.

The Nurse also speaks of moderation and excess—a Greek common-place, to be sure, but she does so using language derived from contemporary discussions of regimen:

βιότου δ' ἀτρεκεῖς ἐπιτηδεύσεις
φασὶ σφάλλειν πλέον ἢ τέρπειν
τῇ θ' ὑγείᾳ μᾶλλον πολεμεῖν.
οὕτω τὸ λίαν ἧσσον ἐπαινῶ
τοῦ μηδὲν ἄγαν·
καὶ ξυμφήσουσι σοφοί μοι.   (261–266)

They say that excessive regimen brings failure more than satisfaction and is inimical to health. Thus I praise excess less than the principle of nothing-in-excess; and the wise agree with me.

In this passage, the Nurse asserts the negative effects of strict regimen on health. The notion of regimen is conveyed by the expression *atrekeis epitêdeuseis*. This expression finds a parallel in the phrase δίαιτα ἀτρεκής used by the author of the Hippocratic treatise *Mochlichon* to denote a strict, curative regimen (42.21). The word *atrekês* is in fact rare in tragedy, although rather common in the Corpus. The noun *epitêdeusis* occurs only once in the Corpus, in the treatise *Regimen* (1.27.9), where it is a synonym for *diaita*; it is only slightly more common in tragedy. However, the related noun *epitêdeuma* does appear six times in the Corpus.[24] *Diaita* is the more standard word for regimen in medical texts. In tragedy, however, *diaita* does not normally have these medical overtones: it simply refers to food eaten at a meal.[25] Thus, even if *epitêdeusis* is the less common word for regimen in the Corpus, it is a word that clearly conveys the idea of 'regimen' (as opposed to 'food' or 'meal') when placed in a tragic context. The Nurse's use of the expression to signify standards or rules for living thus gestures to her interest in rationalist medical ideas. However, the Nurse, in arguing that one should not maintain strict adherence to a daily regimen, refutes the idea of regimen with an appeal to the notion of *mêden agan*, nothing-in-excess. She asserts that, according to what the unidentified 'they' say (*phasi*), a strict regimen 'fails rather than brings pleasure' and that it 'fights with health.' Yet those habits of healthy living which Greek healers tried to systematize into a 'regimen' were in fact based on the

---

[24] Cf., e.g., *Vet. Med.* 20.17, *Reg.* 1.27.5, *Epid.* 1.23.8
[25] Euripides fr. 917 Nauck-Snell (quoted above in the Introduction) provides the exception; in the explicitly medical context of the fragment, he speaks of the *diaitai* of the city dwellers.

common Greek principle of moderation. The healthy must maintain
the most balanced, consistent and moderate of habits if they are to
retain their health.[26] It is rather the sick who must engage in excessive
diets (e.g., liquid diets, barley water diets, 'weak' food diets) in order to
counteract the excessiveness of the disease.[27] The areas in which healers
prescribed moderation included not only nourishment and exercise,
but also drinking and sexual activity. Thus, it is ironic that the Nurse
rejects the idea of strict regimen even as she argues for moderation.
She appeals to an unnamed group of wise 'they's as her authority in
this matter, but here, as in other places, the Nurse seems to combine
different ethical principles into her own special brand of pragmatic
morality.

The audience has been told the nature of Phaedra's illness by Aphrodite in the prologue. But, as Aphrodite emphasizes, no one in the
house understands her disease. In the first part of the play, we follow
the efforts of the Nurse and the chorus to discover the specific nature
of the disease. The idea that one must be able to classify a disease and
distinguish it from other diseases in order to treat it is an important
aspect of fifth-century medicine.[28] The chorus complains at 269 that
Phaedra's disease is ἄσημα ('without signs'): although these women
know that she is sick, they see no symptoms or signs by which they
can diagnose and classify the disease. Questioned by the chorus, the

---

[26] Foucault (1985) analyzes the Hippocratic regimental strictures in the course of his
discussion on the Greek 'aesthetics of experience' (12). Particularly in Part Two, on
'Dietetics,' he explores the dynamics of bodily intake and bodily expenditure in the
Hippocratic Corpus, Plato and Diocles.

[27] It is true that the healthy were governed in such systems by a sort of extreme:
an extreme moderation. The detailed regimen prescribed by later healers such as
Diocles of Carystus shows the extremes to which such ideas could lead, even when
treating healthy individuals. Indeed, in order to achieve health under the care of these
regimen-oriented healers, one would no doubt have to devote one's entire life to the
maintenance of one's physical well-being. The difficulty of attending so carefully to
a daily regimen is recognized by the author of *Regimen*, who divides *Regimen* 3 into
two sections, one dealing with general principles of regimen for the mass of men, and
the other giving very detailed information to those who have the time to devote large
amounts of time and energy to the care of their bodies: see *Reg.* 3.69. Plato criticizes
the regimen movement for excessive devotion to the body and too little attention to
the soul; the soul, in Plato's view, should take priority. For Diocles, see Van der Eijk
(2000–2001); on Plato's views of dietetics, see Wöhrle (1990) 122–149.

[28] Although some healers are accused of misunderstanding the principles of classification: the author of *Regimen in Acute Diseases* criticizes the authors of *Knidiai Gnômai* for
giving different names to every morbid condition, regardless of whether this condition
is merely a variation on a disease already known (*Reg. Acut.* 3).

Nurse explains that Phaedra has thus far resisted her efforts to elicit enough information on which to base a diagnosis (271). She describes the history of the illness: Phaedra has not eaten for three days (275);[29] no, she is not under a delusion of the mind (ὑπ' ἄτης, 276) but is deliberately abstaining from food in an effort to expel life (εἰς ἀπόστασιν βιοῦ, 277). Again we see Euripides' effective use of medical language: normally, *apostasis* refers to the process of expelling disease from the body in order to restore health and maintain life;[30] yet, as Phaedra will soon explain, she has discovered that death alone can cure her disease. Thus, she acts to expel life itself from her body. The Nurse, however, is determined to find another remedy; to do so, she must know the cause of the disease.

The Nurse prides herself on her abilities as a healer—after all, she has perceived Phaedra's disease when Theseus, her own husband, could not. Of course, the Nurse is forced to admit that it is Theseus' absence rather than his lack of acuity which has prevented him from noticing the problem. This short exchange regarding Theseus (278–281) and the ensuing speech by the Nurse (284–310) touch upon a problematic issue in contemporary culture and especially in medicine: the relationship between women and men and more specifically the dynamics between women and their male healers. The chorus indicates that Phaedra's condition is bad enough that her husband should notice it, although she has attempted to conceal it from him. The fact that she should wish to hide an illness from her husband at all seems to engender no surprise among the women, however. Furthermore, in the speech that follows the chorus' questioning, the Nurse makes a distinction between illnesses that can be discussed among and remedied by women alone (293–294) and those which can admit a male healer's attention (295–296). The exposure of the respectable woman's body to the masculine gaze was notionally restricted to very particular circumstances in Athenian society. Women's access to healers—certainly to male healers—would have been regulated by their *kyrioi* (legal guardians). It is unclear to what extent, if any, women were unclothed when examined by a healer. Whether or not she was seen

---

[29] Perhaps this mention of the period of three days is meant to signify to the audience that the onset of a *krisis* is at hand; although healers disagree over whether a *krisis* occurs on even days or odd days, the third and fourth day (as well as the seventh day) often figure in their discussions. On critical days, see more below in section e.

[30] A more extensive discussion of *apostasis* can be found in Part II, pp. 125–128.

nude or even touched by the *iatros*,[31] the introduction of this exceptional, unrelated male into the women's quarters was occasioned only
by the intrusion of disease into the woman's body. In her vulnerable
condition, subjected to disease and to the examination of a man who
was not her husband, a Greek woman would then have to follow the
prescriptions advised by the healer, presumably in consultation with
her *kyrios*. On the other hand, as the work of medical anthropologists
has demonstrated, the proposed remedies would only be acceptable
and indeed effective if they conformed to the belief system held by
the woman and her family.[32] When selecting healers for a woman, it
is possible that Greek men would have trusted more in the diagnoses
and prescriptions of male *iatroi* than in the work of women, who were
difficult to trust.

Euripides has the Nurse suggest that the 'unspeakable' (ἀπορρή-
τοι, 293) diseases could be treated by women alone—otherwise a man
might do it. Thus, he has her imply, women might learn of these hidden
things unspeakable in the more public space of men.[33] Greek male writ-

---

[31] This knotty problem of interactions between male healers and female patients is
discussed by Lloyd (1983) 70–76; Lloyd points to evidence in *Diseases of Women 1* and *Barren Women* where either a female attendant or the patient herself do the actual touching;
on the other hand, he argues that 'there are enough texts that point unambiguously to
the personal intervention of the male healer to establish that female internal examina-
tions were not carried out solely by females' (72); on pp. 72–73 with note 55, he gives
examples, also from gynecological texts (*Diseases of Women 1, Nature of Women*), which he
argues provide the healer's male colleagues with 'explicit instructions on how they are
to conduct an examination and on what they should expect to find when they do so'
(72). Scholars continue to discuss whether such instructions are in fact only theoretical in nature (given the fact that what the healers say they have seen or experienced
often seems quite impossible). For Hippocratic accounts of interactions with female
patients, see also Dean-Jones (1995) and King (1998) 44–49. Galen (*On Prognosis* 8.100–
116 Nutton = *De praenotinone ad Posthumum* 14.641–647 Kühn) describes the efforts of
the wife of Flavius Boethus to hide her problems from a male doctor: ashamed of her
menstrual difficulties, she chose to consult midwives instead. Only when she did not
improve did her husband call upon *iatroi* (among whom was Galen himself). The story
shows both the reticence towards male healers that may have been typical of women
and also different levels of control over health care. On this story, see King (1998)
170.
[32] On the importance of cultural beliefs in the effectiveness of a medical system, see
the fundamental work of Kleinman (1980); for the relationship between cultural beliefs
and the effectiveness of Hippocratic medicine, see King (1998) 22, 114, 116–126, 154–156
and, in many ways, *passim*.
[33] In *Andromache*, Euripides again suggests both the privacy of women's diseases and
the conversations about these diseases that women have among themselves; moreover,
he again suggests that women desire to hide their diseases because these diseases
reveal women's immoral natures. When Hermione castigates her sex for their behavior

ers occasionally indicate their belief that women dislike or reject *iatroi* because women have something to hide.[34] The Nurse's words exclude men from knowledge of women's hidden diseases, exactly as men would expect. More significantly, however, Phaedra herself believes that her disease is something that must not be communicated at all; if it is to be communicated, such communication should be confined to the circle of women. The disease must remain hidden, for its revelation would mean shame and loss of honor for her, a circumstance that she contends would render her life unlivable. Indeed, to disclose the disease in speech is to strengthen its power and to make it infectious—the disclosure results in two deaths and the destruction of a family. Thus, we should note that, as Phaedra points out to the Nurse at 352, she herself never says the name Hippolytus, which she equates with her disease. The Nurse, by contrast, despite the distinctions she has made between the women and the male healers, fails to understand the danger of speaking the name of the disease and of communicating it to men. By giving the disease a name, a classification, an existence in language, and by speaking this name outside the company of women, she gives it the power to destroy both Phaedra and Hippolytus and she loses any power to cure it.

The play's use of what I have argued are medical ideas also provides us with evidence as to possible distinctions perceived in this period between medical science, magic, and religion. The Nurse assumes that Phaedra can explain what her problem is, or at least can identify her

---

'behind closed doors' (ὑγιὲς γὰρ οὐδὲν αἱ θύραθεν εἴσοδοι / δμῶσιν γυναικῶν, ἀλλὰ πολλὰ καὶ κακά, 952–953: 'For the entrances of women behind the door accomplish nothing healthy, but rather many evil things'), the chorus agrees, but submits that women ought not to reveal the bad nature of these 'women's diseases' in public: συγγνωστὰ μέν νυν σοὶ τάδ᾽, ἀλλ᾽ ὅμως χρεὼν / κοσμεῖν γυναῖκας τὰς γυναικείας νόσους (955–956: 'It is understandable that you would say these things, but nevertheless it is necessary that women should present women's diseases in a decent light'). The term γυναικεῖα νοσήματα occurs in the Hippocratic Corpus (cf. *Nat. Puer.* 15.6, 58.22; *Morb.* 4.57.6, 121.1; *Steril.* 113) as does the term γυναικεῖαι νοῦσοι (*Genit.* 4.47).

Goff (1990: 1–2) interprets the Nurse's speech at 293–296 as part of a larger concern in the play: the interplay of speech and silence with gender roles and spatial arrangements; on its thematic significance, cf. also McClure (1999) 125–127.

[34] Witness Galen's story about diagnosing love-sickness in a married woman patient (the wife of Justus) by detecting a change in her pulse rate whenever the name of the actor Pylades was mentioned (*On Prognosis* 6.100–102 Nutton = *De praenotione ad Posthumum* 14.631–634 Kühn). On the deceitfulness of women and their bodies, and the significance of this for the Hippocratic *iatroi*, see King (1998) 45–53 (who also discusses the passage in *Hippolytus* briefly on p. 47)

pain; moreover, as I have already argued, she frequently makes use
of language and ideas common in medical circles. Yet at 236–238,
she attributes Phaedra's delirious fantasies to the attack of some god
whose identity can only be discovered through prophecy; at 346, she
announces that she herself is no prophet (μάντις) and cannot therefore fathom invisible or unclear things (τἀφανῆ). Phaedra's disease has
been *asêma* (269): no symptoms have appeared which might signify the
underlying disease. In the absence of physical, visible signs, science has
no power to interpret. In contrast to the aspirations of the healers by
whom she seems to be inspired, the Nurse admits she is no prophet,
admits that she cannot understand things which are not clear. Her lack
of ability to know the past, understand the present, and most impor-
tantly, predict the outcome of the situation is in fact a commentary
on her incompetence as a healer. Once the nature of the disease has
been revealed in speech (and the Nurse has recovered from her shock
upon learning the truth), she draws upon examples of divine behavior
(451–458) in order to bolster her argument that Phaedra has not acted
wrongly by falling in love with Hippolytus; after all, Aphrodite herself,
to whose irresistible force even Zeus must bow, is responsible for Phaedra's plight. Yet the remedy she proposes to resolve Phaedra's situation
looks neither to fifth-century medical procedures nor to traditional religious methods of prayer and sacrifice for its justification. Instead, the
Nurse's remedy belongs to the realm of magic: at 478, she mentions
ἐπῳδαὶ καὶ λόγοι θελκτήριοι ('incantations and words of enchantment');
at 509, she speaks of φίλτρα … θελκτήρια ('love potions' or 'potions
of enchantment') which require such clearly magical ingredients as
hair from the beloved's head or some piece of his/her clothing (514).
None of these remedies are ever suggested in the Hippocratic Corpus—
indeed, these are exactly the sort of treatments the rationalist healer is
determined to condemn and avoid.[35] As Charles Segal points out, the
Nurse at this point switches from the allopathic methods espoused by

---

[35] As Ann Hanson argues, the recipes for the drug therapies in the Hippocratic
Corpus were drawn no doubt from age-old recipes long used in traditional ('folk')
medicine. It was the role of the rationalist healer to place these therapies into a
new, more sophisticated context, and to account in some way for their effectiveness.
See Hanson (1991) esp. 79–87 (on pessaries and odor therapies). In the light of her
arguments, I should perhaps call Hippocratic drug therapy 'rationalized' rather than
'rationalist.' It is also important to note that the Hippocratic Corpus is not entirely
'purged' of the instruments that are said to be magical; see, e.g., Hanson's discussion of
the uterine amulets employed in Greek medicine (1995).

most Hippocratics to the homeopathic methods so common in magic.[36] The Nurse's attempt to use magical potions or spells marks her as an incompetent rationalist: as the author of *On the Sacred Disease* stresses (1.10–12), only charlatans and sorcerers would resort to such things.[37]

After her disastrous attempt to find a cure in Hippolytus himself, the Nurse faces the enraged Phaedra and tries to justify her actions. Having behaved irrationally,[38] she now uses the language of Hippocratic medicine in her defense. Phaedra's judgment (διάγνωσις) is wrong, she argues in 696, because it has been overwhelmed by biting pain (δάκνον). Patients cannot diagnose their own illnesses because they are in pain and cannot see the whole situation—thus, the need for the objective gaze of the healer. Now the Nurse no longer speaks of *philtra thelktêria*, but instead returns to the neutral term *pharmaka* (699).[39] She insists she was acting with the best intentions, but admits she was not very successful or *sôphrôn* (704). Success would have placed her among the *sophoi* (700), a group to which she had earlier claimed to belong (we recall that at line 266 the *sophoi* agreed with *her*). The Nurse insists she is not a deliberately bad healer, just an incompetent one. She would like to have another try (705).

---

[36] Segal (1992) 436. It should be stressed that homeopathic remedies are not foreign to the Hippocratic Corpus, so it is not on this criterion alone that the Nurse should be seen as diverging from rationalistic practices. Rather it is the combination of homeopathic methods and the actual contents of the remedies (spells, hair, clothing) that mark the new direction of her approach. On homeopathy and allopathy, see more in Part II, pp. 115–121.

[37] For Hippocratic 'attacks' on magic, see discussion in Lloyd (1979) 15–29; see also Laskaris (2002), who rightly stresses the rhetorical nature of these attacks.

[38] Apart from her stated intention to use magical remedies, how could she possibly think that the chaste and rigid Hippolytus, of all people, would be sympathetic to Phaedra's plight?

[39] Neutral in the sense that the word *pharmakon* is to be found in both medical and magical texts, and also in the sense that a *pharmakon* is not of necessity a remedy: it can also be a poison. The term is flexible, and its interpretation depends heavily on context: pharmacological substances operate on a continuum: they can be helpful or harmful depending on the amount of the substance used and the manner of application. See Harig (1977). In discussing the various theories behind Mithridates' notorious resistance to poison, Harig points out that Greeks seem to have considered poison an inappropriately strong dosage of a substance which, when appropriately administered, could be a useful curative. Cf. also Artelt (1937) 94–96. On the use of the term *pharmakon* and its application in spheres of activity which we consider separate today, see Scarborough (1991). Scarborough warns against making easy distinctions between magical, religious, and medical usages of *pharmaka*; see esp. 141–145, 150–151, 161–163. For a discussion on the term *pharmakon* as a metaphor for the 'dangerous instability' of language in *Hippolytus*, see Goff (1990) 48–54.

Phaedra will have none of it. Incredulous that the Nurse persists, even after having 'wounded' (τρώσασαν, 703) her, she commands her to 'stop talking' (706). Talking has thus far in the play brought nothing but fresh pain. Dismissing the Nurse to tend to her own affairs, Phaedra announces that she will cure herself: ἐγὼ δὲ τἀμὰ θήσομαι καλῶς (709). As Barrett points out, these words echo those of the Nurse just before she went to tell Hippolytus of Phaedra's love (521). Phaedra's cure for herself will in fact be an 'incurable evil' (ἀνήκεστον κακόν, 722): death. Nevertheless, Phaedra, while dying to preserve her good name, at the same time wishes to hurt Hippolytus. Now it is she who uses the word *nosos* not in the sense of 'love-sickness' but in a more general sense that embraces both physical suffering and mental distress (730). In becoming the healer of her own troubles, Phaedra learns to spread disease and Hippolytus will learn to suffer from it.

Euripides' work thus shows us how the argument about suffering of healers advanced by *Breaths*' author can become unconvincing when placed in the context of an actual illness and moreover on the lips of an amoral practitioner. The Nurse persuades Phaedra not by using a consistent line of reasoning or a compelling moral argument; instead, she wears her out with different proposals. Furthermore, she ultimately resorts to deceitful practices in order to heal her patient. Her rhetoric may convince the weakened and anguished Phaedra, but it does not have the same effect on the audience, which is surely meant to reject the practices and prescriptions of the Nurse. However, the author of *Breaths* is more sophisticated in his rhetoric than the Nurse: he presents his argument in terms much more acceptable to a fifth-century audience, as he maintains and sets the mere private suffering of the healer against what he achieves, common good. Furthermore, he acknowledges that the healer's suffering relieves the patient from the 'greatest evils' (*megistôn kakôn*). Hence, he does not appear to suggest that the healer suffers *more* than the patient, but rather that he suffers some pain from unpleasant visual and tactile stimuli—certainly not more painful than the disease suffered by the patient. By setting the common good ahead of his personal comfort, the healer is certainly engaging in behavior endorsed time and again elsewhere in Greek literature, especially in the classical period.

The author of *Breaths* grants to the healer a powerful role, one which takes on the primary responsibility of the struggle against the disease; his position contrasts, as I have said, with that of some other authors in the Corpus, such as that of *Epidemics* i, who argues that the healer's role is subordinate to that of both the *technê* and the patient. Furthermore, critiques of medical practice tend to focus on the incompetence of the healer rather than on the limits of the *technê*. Even the author of *Breaths* admits that there is such a thing as a bad healer, but he nonetheless represents the relationship of the healer to the *technê* as horizontal rather than vertical when he describes the poor healer as removed from the *technê*: ἰητρικὴ γάρ ἐστιν ἀφαίρεσις καὶ πρόσθεσις, ἀφαίρεσις μὲν τῶν πλεοναζόντων, πρόσθεσις δὲ τῶν ἐλλειπόντων· ὁ δὲ τοῦτ᾽ ἄριστα ποιέων ἄριστος ἰητρός· ὁ δὲ τούτου πλεῖστον ἀπολείφθεὶς πλεῖστον ἀπελείφθη τῆς τέχνης (1.5: 'for medicine is addition and subtraction, subtraction of what is excessive and addition of what is lacking; the best healer is the one who does this best, whereas the one who is most removed from this is also most removed from the *technê*'). The author of the *Law* uses a striking image to describe poor healers when he compares them to extras ('masks') in a tragedy, who wear costumes and masks, but are nonetheless not actors: ὁμοιότατοι γάρ εἰσιν οἱ τοιοίδε τοῖσι παρεισαγομένοισι προσώποισιν ἐν τῆσι τραγῳδίῃσιν· ὡς γὰρ ἐκεῖνοι σχῆμα μὲν καὶ στολὴν καὶ πρόσωπον ὑποκριτοῦ ἔχουσιν, οὐκ εἰσὶ δὲ ὑποκριταί, οὕτω καὶ ἰητροί, φήμῃ μὲν πολλοί, ἔργῳ δὲ πάγχυ βαιοί (1: 'Most similar are such men to "masks" brought on in tragedies; for while they have the appearance, dress and mask of an actor, they are not actors. Thus also with healers: many exist in reputation, but very few in reality'). Extras are subordinate and assistant to the actors in a tragedy, and, though they may look like the real thing, they do not have access to the true *technê* of acting. Like actors, true healers match appearance and reality: they embody the *technê*. The relationship of the healer to the *technê* was clearly an issue under dispute among the writers of the Corpus: was the relationship horizontal or vertical, was the healer master or servant? How was one to distinguish between the true healer and the charlatan? Who (or what) is ultimately responsible for fighting the disease? Once again, it is useful to observe the cultural context in which these discussions are taking place. Let us turn once again to Euripides, to examine the issue of power assigned to wielders of *technê*.

Let us begin with characters who are subordinate in status—but not necessarily in dramatic function—to the protagonists of the play. We have in fact already considered one such character, the Nurse in *Hippolytus*, who applies her wisdom so disastrously. Similar to the Nurse is the Old Man in *Ion* as he acts upon the hopes and fears of Creousa. These confidante characters are characterized by a loyalty to their respective mistresses that is both shortsighted and monocular; thus it is not surprising that their attempts at healing should be characterized by incompetence. It is their task to help their superior when she is in trouble, but, because they have limited authority (and perhaps limited intelligence), they can do little against the larger forces arrayed against the protagonist. Sadly, their perspective is narrower than that of the tragic sufferer and their suggested solutions, well intentioned as they are, prove disastrous. The Nurse acts against Phaedra's (stated) will in an attempt to cure her of her disease; unfortunately, her action leads to Phaedra's death by suicide. But her role, which is so significant in many ways to the action of the plot, is ultimately forgotten in the play's resolution: at stake in *Hippolytus* is not the ethics of the Nurse, but rather those of Phaedra, Theseus and Hippolytus.[40] Moreover, as Aphrodite explains, Phaedra is but an instrument in her designs against Hippolytus—and thus, presumably, the Nurse's role in the whole scheme is all the more incidental. If we can compare her to the figures discussed in the *Law*, the Nurse is a healer in rhetorical dress only. But if the Nurse fails to heal, she is nonetheless a powerful force in the development of the play—no extra is she. The Old Man is the first to suggest the murder of Ion, but fortunately he bungles his part of the job (and of course, had he not, the *Ion* might have ended more like *Hippolytus*, with Creousa coming to the terrible realization that she has just had her son killed, rather than the merely distressing thought that she has almost done so). There are indeed significant differences between the parts played by these old servants. The reasons for these differences lie not only in the mythical traditions themselves, which call for Ion to live and Phaedra to die, but also in the relationship presented between mistress and servant. The Nurse in *Hippolytus* is forceful and opinionated, while Phaedra is weakened by illness and consumed by shame. By contrast, the Old Man is weak and fragile, needing Creousa's help as much as she needs his, and they work in

---

[40] In his important and persuasive discussion of elite and non-elite in tragedy (and in Athens), Griffith (1995) argues that it is an essential feature of tragedy that the chorus and the 'minor' characters *survive* and that furthermore, however aware they are of the suffering of the elite protagonists, these characters remain 'immune from the adverse "changes of fortune" that mark the kinds of tragic action' (122). This reinforces a certain ideology, argues Griffith, in which the elite risk the most and therefore are culturally and politically valuable. The Nurse does take more risks and interfere more than many non-elite characters in tragedy, but she also survives to fade without further mention from the action of the play.

tandem to dévise and execute an attack on Ion. But it is in fact the Old Man who takes the lead in diagnosing the situation and suggesting appropriate remedies.

c. Ion: *Malpractice suits*

Ion presents the limitations of human deduction and human planning even as it startles us by presenting the limitations of divine planning as well. In a world where even the god of prophecy fails to predict the future accurately, it is perhaps not surprising that humans would have such trouble understanding the past and foretelling what is to come. We are given three accounts of Ion's conception in the play: two are at least plausible when judged according to the norms of human behavior; the remaining one, which involves direct divine participation, seems far more incredible, but is in fact the true story. Furthermore, the explanations proffered by Xuthus and Ion (545–556), on the one hand, and by the Old Man (813–829), on the other, both deny Creousa her rightful role in the generative process; moreover, the pain of this public exclusion is added to her private, secret pain, the pain of Apollo's rape and subsequent abandonment of her and her child. Creousa comes to Delphi seeking a cure for this private pain—she calls herself 'sick' (νοσοῦσα) at 320—as well as for the more open 'disease' of her infertility. Creousa's need for secrecy places her in a peculiar situation: she has been deemed infertile (a great failing in any Greek woman) yet she cannot reveal the proof of her fertility (both because of her own shame and because she no longer has the child as evidence).[41] Her isolation is only increased by her exclusion from any role in producing Ion; with this

---

[41] Infertility is usually perceived to be a woman's problem in ancient Greece: male seed ought, it seems, to bear fruit if it finds the right soil in which to grow. This remains true whether the model of conception is based on the existence of both male and female seed *vel sim.* (this is the more common model, to which the Hippocratics generally ascribed) or the model in which the male alone provides seed (most prominent in Aristotle, but found earlier, perhaps most famously in Aesch. *Eum.* 658–666). On Hippocratic and Aristotelian understandings of male and female roles in conception, see the extensive discussion in Dean-Jones (1994) ch. 3. Hanson (1990: 327) remarks that 'the notion that the gods expect their every violation of a female to bear fruit was a topos [in note 90, she cites Hesiod, *Gyn. Cat.* fr. 31 Merkelbach-West and Euripides, fr. 73a Snell], and the many therapies in the *Corpus* which attempt to cure sterility in women strongly suggest that the Greek man also felt that his lovemaking should result in a child, unless the reproductive apparatus of his partner was defective.'

comes of course an exclusion from any part or significance in the ruling dynasty of Athens. In the first part of the scene in which Creousa
and the Old Man learn of Ion's new position, Creousa remains in pain
and isolated because of her refusal to disclose her own history; however,
after she has revealed her private suffering, she is able to look for a cure.
She finds one in the use of her family's drugs to kill Ion: if she cannot
participate in generation, then she will at least wreak destruction.

The interactions between Creousa and the Old Man during their
scene together parallel the larger situation in which Creousa's central
position in the Athenian polis is reduced to a peripheral one. Moreover,
the language of disease and medicine is frequently called upon to
express these dynamics. Thus, as the two characters enter, the Old Man
is depicted as weak and aged, and, moreover, very much in need of
Creousa's assistance. Her authority and power is made manifest by his
request that she act as the 'healer of his old age' (739–740). The Old
Man goes on to insist that his mind is still swift even if his feet are slow
(742); the next four verses indicate that he is physically disabled, both in
strength of body and, more significantly, in the power of his eyesight:

Κρέουσα. βάκτρῳ δ' ἐρείδου· περιφερὴς στίβος χθονός.
Πρεσβύτης. καὶ τοῦτο τυφλόν, ὅταν βλέπω βραχύ.
Κρέουσα. ὀρθῶς ἔλεξας· ἀλλὰ μὴ παρῇς κόπῳ.
Πρεσβύτης. οὔκουν ἑκών γε· τοῦ δ' ἀπόντος οὐ κρατῶ.   (743–746)

Creousa. Lean on your staff: be watchful of the track on the ground.
Old Man. This too is blind business, when I see a short distance.
Creousa. You have spoken rightly: but don't give in to weariness.
Old Man. Not willingly, at any rate: but I don't have control over what
    is absent.

Touchingly concerned for the Old Man's welfare, Creousa is soon faced
with her own loss, however—not of her physical powers, but of her
authority and even of her identity. The chorus' mournful greetings indicate to her that something is wrong (she can read these verbal signs):
she asks, ἀλλ' ἦ τι θεσφάτοισι δεσποτῶν νοσεῖ; (755: 'Is something disordered in the oracles for the masters?'). The word *nosei* is telling: it means
not just 'be wrong' but 'be in disorder' or 'be abnormal.'[42] Creousa's

---

[42] In contrast to the many instances of the noun *nosos* in archaic literature, the verb
noseô does not appear until well into the classical period (the first extant citation is at
Soph. *Aias* 635). The word does have a wide semantic range, but nevertheless retains its
close association with disease. There were plenty of other verbs available to Euripides
with which to express a more general sense of 'be wrong' without the connotation of
disease. On the history of the word *nosos* and its cognates, see Preiser (1976).

use of the word anticipates the news which is to come, news which means the total reversal of the traditional Athenian order. Ion himself had earlier stated that he would suffer from 'two diseases' (δύο νόσω) in Athens: a foreign father and an illegitimate birth (591–592). Indeed, in Euripides' day, such a person could lay no claim to Athenian citizenship. Furthermore, Ion's newly acquired position in the ruling family of Athens undercuts the importance of the Athenian claim to autochthony, so central to their sense of identity, it circumvents the need for Athenian parentage, and it negates the need for female participation in the establishment of Athenian identity. This is public disorder indeed.[43]

Creousa reacts to the news of the oracle not only with emotional anguish but also with physical pain: διανταῖος ἔτυπεν ὀδύνα με πλευ- / μόνων τῶνδ' ἔσω (767–768: 'deep pain has struck me in my chest'). Just as Apollo has caused her pain and distress when he had raped her years earlier, so now the words of his oracle strike pain into her breast. As we have seen above, of all the words for pain in Greek, *odynê* would seem to have the most physical connotations.[44] In the lines that follow the initial disclosure of the chorus, Creousa seems to be increasingly overcome with pain. Creousa can only respond to each fresh piece of news, giving further expression to her own personal feelings, while the Old Man solicits all the additional information. Reversing their earlier postures of 'healer' and 'patient,' the Old Man now tries to take on the role of helper and comforter;[45] for the next eighty lines or so (769–843), it is he who interprets, analyzes, suggests, and soothes.

The Old Man urges Creousa not to groan before they have heard the whole of the matter. To him, as an Athenian resentful of foreign intrusion, the essential matter to be determined is whether Xuthus shares in this disaster (*symphora*) or whether Creousa is to suffer alone (771–772). Unaware of the double nature of Creousa's pain, he sees the situation as salvageable only if Xuthus suffers too. When the chorus explains that Xuthus has been given the young temple attendant as a son (794–795), Creousa bursts out with the wish that she might escape this place, such is the pain she suffers (796–799). She then falls silent for the next fifty lines (until 859 when she begins her monody) and the Old Man begins his analysis of the situation.

---

[43] For more detailed discussion of the political implications of the play and the significance of Creousa's position for Athens, see Loraux (1981) and Saxonhouse (1992).

[44] See above (notes 16 and 17).

[45] The reversal is also discussed by Lee *ad* 808.

Although the Old Man may have argued that one should not leap to
conclusions before obtaining all the facts, he himself is quick to turn to
broad speculation as he reconstructs—incorrectly—the course of events
leading up to Xuthus' sudden acquisition of an adolescent son (813–
829). Significantly, despite his belief in the miraculous autochthony of
the Athenians, the Old Man offers here a very prosaic account of Ion's
begetting. Just as Ion insisted on finding a non-miraculous explanation
for his newfound position, so, too, the Old Man formulates an explanation that has no miraculous underpinnings. We should note that Ion
and Xuthus[46] come up with the more credible story considering Ion's
age; yet the main impetus for both these accounts seems to be that
'rational' explanations are more desirable and more believable than
explanations which require belief in divine intervention or supernatural
forces of some kind. Oracles, it appears, are felt to be only divine explanations of natural events; they are not meant to suggest direct divine
involvement.

The Old Man does not look at the evidence with his own eyes, he
does not examine the individuals involved, he relies on the words of
the chorus and his own 'quick mind' to concoct a history for Ion.
Moreover, concerned as he is with his own sense of betrayal, he fails
to see the deeper nature of Creousa's suffering. It is only after her long
monody, in which a 'storehouse of evils' is disclosed (923–924), that the
Old Man turns his attention to examining more closely the nature of
Creousa's distress (925–933). In the sequence following the monody, the
focus alters from discussing the disease from which 'we' suffer (cf. 808)
to considering the pain that affects Creousa alone, a change from
empathy to sympathy. Now the concern is for Creousa's secret *nosos*,
her private suffering, unnoticed by the Old Man until now because a
wave of troubles was overwhelming his mind (927). As she begins to
reveal the hidden details of her past in a stichomythic exchange, the
Old Man claims to have in fact discerned her *nosos* many years earlier:

> Πρεσβύτης. ὦ θύγατερ, ἆρ᾽ ἦν ταῦθ᾽ ἅ γ᾽ ἠσθόμην ἐγώ;
> Κρέουσα. οὐκ οἶδ᾽· ἀληθῆ δ᾽ εἰ λέγεις φαίημεν ἄν.
> Πρεσβύτης. νόσον κρυφαίαν ἡνίκ᾽ ἔστενες λάθραι.   (942–944)

> Old Man. Oh daughter, was it this then that I perceived?
> Creousa. I don't know: but if you speak truthfully, we would admit it.
> Old Man. When you were groaning in secret over a hidden disease.

---

[46] Xuthus has in fact dismissed the possibility of autochthony with the words οὐ
πέδον τίκτει τέκνα (542: 'the ground does not bear children').

Now Creousa makes manifest to the chorus and the Old Man her long concealed and painful story (τότ' ἦν ἃ νῦν σοι φανερὰ σημαίνω κακά, 945: 'those were the troubles then which I am revealing to you now'). In these lines of revelation, Euripides has used words which combine to bring out the medical undertones of the scene: Creousa's hidden disease is now exposed through signification (*sêmainô*), a process of signification begun by her lamentation and now completed by her explanation. The treatise *Regimen* explains that diseases do not appear at once (εὐθέως), but gather themselves together little by little (κατὰ μίκρον) before making a sudden appearance; the good healer will nonetheless notice the suffering of the patient 'before the health in the person is mastered by the disease' (πρὶν οὖν κρατεῖσθαι ἐν τῷ ἀνθρώπῳ τὸ ὑγιὲς ὑπὸ τοῦ νοσεροῦ) and intervene appropriately to maintain or restore health (1.2). The Old Man may have noticed her disease in the past, but he was not able to diagnose it further nor intervene before it mastered her; she had concealed the symptoms too well.

Creousa is now in utter despair over her situation. She sees no way to combat the betrayal of Apollo or of her husband (ἀπορία τὸ δυστυχεῖν, 971). But the Old Man offers some possible if objectionable remedies (972–977). Creousa rejects the idea of burning the temple or of killing her husband, but the murder of Ion she is willing to consider. Once again, the Old Man plays the role of instigator as he suggests possible methods for killing Ion (980–983). When Creousa rejects both of his suggestions, the Old Man, unable to think of any other plan, abandons his role of counselor and hands over the reins to Creousa: μοι, κακίζῃ· φέρε, σύ νυν βούλευέ τι (984: 'alas, you are cowardly; but come, you contrive something now').[47] It is Creousa who must now draw upon the strength of her extraordinary ancestry as she contrives a way to deal with the encroaching outsider. She turns to the *pharmaka* that her father had given her, the blood of the Gorgon containing both harmful and healing powers.[48] One might argue that these *pharmaka*,

---

[47] Lee *ad* 971 observes that 'the motif of adviser and advised changing places is recurrent in Euripidean plotting scenes' and compares *Hel.* 1035ff. and 1049ff. and *IT* 1017ff. and 1029ff.

[48] The conception of blood in the ancient world is a story in itself. Blood is a substance both essential and dangerous: e.g., women must menstruate every month as a sign of their health and fertility, yet it is during this very period that they are considered a source of pollution; blood sacrifice is a necessary element in the ritual purification of homicides. However, blood rarely comes up as an ingredient in healing remedies provided in the Hippocratic Corpus. The degree to which a menstruating women was a source of pollution is a problematic issue in current scholarship: von

with their origins in the mythical world of Gorgons and such, hardly belong to the view of medicine developing in the fifth century. Yet, as I have said before, we must not be too hasty in dividing rational from non-rational, or medical from magical.[49] While I would not argue that these drugs were produced by rational means, they are to be used in the public setting of a banquet, and they require no magic spells to enforce their power.[50] Moreover, they have been introduced into a context wherein the miraculous has been suppressed and rational forms of explanation and inquiry have been foregrounded. Furthermore, it is surely no accident that Creousa and the Old Man decide that *ios* (1015) would be an effective means of doing away with *Ion*—the pun on Ion's name[51] also suggests the use of a homeopathic remedy: the use of poison to expunge poison. The terms *koilê phlebs* (the hollow vessel, 1011) and *dynamis* (capacity, 1012), prominent in contemporary medical discussions,[52] contribute to the overlapping of medical and magical language in the scene. Finally, the very nature of the *pharmaka*, which stem from the same source but which have two opposing affects, is reminiscent of the paradox, common in Presocratic philosophy, that the same substance which makes sick men well can make well men sick; a similar paradox points out that whereas sickness is bad for the patient, it is good for the healer, whose practice depends upon the existence of

---

Staden (1992), esp. 14, argues that menstrual blood is polluting, whereas Cole (1992) maintains that menstruation *per se* is not always a strong source of pollution. For blood as a source of pollution, see Parker (1983), frequently, but cf., e.g., 55, 230–231, 370–374. King (1998: 88–98) underscores the Hippocratic use of sacrificial imagery to describe menstrual bleeding and argues that the Greeks see menstruation as 'fundamental ... to the maintenance of present order' (98). See also the discussion in Lanata (1967) 45–46, who notes the importance of blood in magic, as part of the magical principle of *similia similibus curantur* (homeopathy). I discuss homeopathy more extensively in Part II, pp. 118–121.

[49] Cf. above (notes 35, 36, 39).

[50] The importance of spells (Gr. *epôidai)* for the correct execution of magic is discussed in Lanata (1967) 46–51.

[51] The derivation of Ion's name remains disputed, but is subject to some discussion in the play; cf. 661–662 for the naming of Ion by Xuthus and 831 (perhaps not genuine) for a pun involving another derivation, 'going' (Ἴων, ἰόντι ...). On the significance of naming Ion in the play, see Zacharia (2003) 125–128, with references to scholarship on Ion's name at 126 n. 102.

[52] Although it must be admitted that these terms are certainly not limited to fifth-century medical discussions—particularly the *koilê phlebs*, which has a long history in Greek anatomical description. For *koilê phlebs* in the Hippocratic Corpus, cf. the description of the vascular system in *Loc. Hom.* 2–3, esp. 3.5, with commentary by Craik *ad loc.* For *dynamis*, see Plamböck (1964).

sick people.⁵³ In *Ion*, the same substance, Gorgon's blood, can harm or help. The two aspects of the substance are distinguished in the course of the scene as originating from different parts of the Gorgon's body. Creousa keeps them separated, pure, unmixed, so that they can maintain their efficacy (1016–1017). Thus, the play incorporates the language of sophisticated medicine into this scene, while at the same time describing events and objects possible only in the world of myth.

These special *pharmaka*, handed down to Creousa through the generations of her family, signify her legitimate position in the clan of Erichthonius—in much the same way as the tokens in the basket will establish Ion's true identity as a member of the same clan. The *pharmaka* restore authority to Creousa as much by their legitimation of her identity as by their power to destroy Ion. The Old Man, for all his loyalty and his eagerness to help, is excluded from that specialized identity; thus, it is perhaps not surprising that he ultimately fails to manipulate the poison successfully. He is proud of his status as an Athenian, an *autochthôn*, but he is not a member of the ruling clan. He believes he possesses a sharp mind; he is certainly quick to find explanations and suggest remedies; he prides himself on his analytical ability, claiming to have noticed Creousa's secret all those many years before. Moreover, it is he who asks most of the questions in the scene, interrogating first the chorus and then Creousa, determined to establish the facts of the situation. Yet he helps Creousa to entirely the wrong conclusion, for Ion is in fact her son, not someone who has gained his position through fictions constructed by Xuthus and Apollo. Again, in suggesting retaliation as a remedy, it is the Old Man who directs Creousa at last against the least culpable of her male opponents. Finally—and fortunately—, he fails in the attempt to poison Ion, but thereafter immediately betrays Creousa (1215–1216), the very person whom he was so eager to help.

The failure of both rationalist explanation and magical potions is essential to the happy outcome of *Ion*, a play in which no one's plans (except for those of the rather oblivious Xuthus) turn out the way they are supposed to. Only the timely arrival of the priestess with Ion's birth tokens in hand achieves the recognition between mother and son. Their joyful reunion thus results from mere chance rather than from planning, anticipation, or analysis. There are many failed rationalists in this play (Apollo, ironically, is one of them); thus, it is significant for

---

⁵³ Cf. Heraclitus DK22 B58 and *Dissoi Logoi* DK90 1 (3).

our understanding of Athenian thinking in this period that the language of disease and medicine finds consistent, albeit limited, employment in *Ion*. Medical methods, influenced by the development of Greek
rationalist thought, help to structure action in the play. Furthermore,
the medical semantics of certain words and phrases overlap with their
magical and religious meanings, creating a linguistic tension that reinforces the tension between the image of the sophisticated Athenians of
the fifth century and the miraculous nature of their autochthonous origins. The scene in which Creousa and the Old Man react to the oracle
exploits attitudes typical of Hippocratic medicine to expose the incompetence of the Old Man. In his attempt to find some remedy against
Creousa's public loss of stature and her private loss of a son so many
years earlier, he unwittingly sets out to kill that very same son; in so
doing, he risks achieving not her health and happiness, but her destruction.

d. Medea: *First, do no harm*

The Old Man in *Ion* is at a remove both from power and from *technê*.
Although a servant of Creousa, he is a poor servant of *technê*. The
Euripidean characters who act or attempt to act as incompetent healers
are often lower in status than their 'patients' and peripheral to the
central conflict of the protagonists: they are devoted only to the health
of their patient and are not interested in larger concerns of the *oikos*
or the *polis*. I would now like to examine a character who has power
because she is an extremely able wielder of *technê*, Medea. As a woman
and barbarian, Medea has little control over her own destiny, but she is
able to compensate for the inferiority assigned to her by Greek culture
through her *sophia*. Medea is no servant of the *technê*—she is its master,
able to use it to help or to harm. Skilled in pharmacology, clever, self-
sufficient, credited with possession of a *technê*—thus far, Medea has all
the desirable characteristics of a good healer. But Medea rarely uses
these skills in a manner compliant with the ethical principles laid down
by physicians in the Hippocratic Corpus. Medea seems to go about
the medical business in an entirely contrary way. Far from using her
expertise to heal, she uses it to deceive, to maim, and to kill. At the
same time, the remedy chosen by Medea is ultimately one from which
she herself suffers; in killing Jason's children, she also kills her own,
and thus chooses to inflict pain upon herself. Of course, her motives in

choosing self-inflicted pain are hardly altruistic: instead, Medea acts in an attempt both to erase the past and to reciprocate the pain that Jason has caused her.

The play indicates in the prologue and in the ensuing discussion between the Nurse and the Paedagogus that Medea is in some way sick. In the early portion of the play, the Nurse plays the role of healer as she describes Medea's condition and gives a diagnosis as to cause: Medea is sick because of Jason's betrayal. The description of Medea's condition recalls and foreshadows portraits of sick characters found in other dramas. Like Aias in Sophocles' *Aias* (323–325), Phaedra in *Hippolytus* (275, 277), and Orestes in *Orestes* (41), she lies, not eating; she wastes away with the time (κεῖται δ' ἄσιτος, σῶμ' ὑφεῖσ' ἀλγηδόσιν,/ τὸν πάντα συντήκουσα δακρύοις χρόνον, 24–25).[54] Yet but for these symptoms, Medea's sickness is of a rather different order than that of these other characters, for Medea is more than usually active in the production of her own illness. She fits the pattern of lying despondent without eating, an action chosen by Phaedra in her determination to die and lamented by Iphis in *Suppliant Women* (1105–1106) as a vision of his grief-stricken old age. Medea too has chosen not to eat; she has chosen to lie prostrate. Yet unlike the enfeebled Phaedra, Medea's passive state belies her active mind. She is an uneasy combination of patient and agent; Jason's actions have caused her to suffer, but her sickness is self-induced. Thus, the Nurse states not that her heart moves or that she is moved by anger, but rather that μήτηρ κινεῖ κραδίαν, κινεῖ δὲ χόλον (98–99: 'she moves her heart, she moves her anger').

---

[54] The interpretation of συντήκω is a problem here. Συντήκω and τήκω in both tragedy and medical writings very often describe the physical 'wasting' of a sick person. But Page argues that in this passage Medea is not wasting physically, but she is rather wasting away the time (χρόνον is after all in the accusative). Yet almost all other Euripidean instances in which συντήκω/τήκω appear in the context of human suffering clearly refer to the decay/wasting of the individual him or herself. Συντήκω: *El.* 240–241; *Or.* 34, 238; *Supp.* 1106; fr. 296 Nauck-Snell. Τήκω: *Med.* 159; *El.* 208, 1209 (Seidler's emendation); *Heraclid.* 645, fr. 908 Nauck-Snell. *IA* 398 (ἐμὲ δὲ συντήξουσι νύκτες … δακρύοις) is the only example which comes close to what Page wants, because although the literal translation is 'the nights will waste me away with tears,' the meaning seems to be 'I shall waste away the nights with tears.' But the order of the Greek doesn't actually *say* that, and I would argue that the suggestion is that *both* the body of the speaker and the nights themselves are included in the wasting away. The association of συντήκω with physical wasting is simply too strong, I think, to avoid this. Thus, although the syntax of the *Medea* passage is clear, I believe that the semantics of the verb συντήκω suggest some involvement of Medea herself in this process of 'wasting.' Mastronarde *ad loc.* finds it an 'odd usage,' as he argues for such a conflation.

Movement in the context of illness is dangerous according to Greek thinking; organs and/or fluids moving around were often held either responsible for, or accessory to, the onset of disease.[55] Furthermore, *cholos* (anger) is the Attic-Ionic form of *cholê* (bile); we can still see the corporal connotation of *cholos* at work in the *Iliad*: Achilles' anger clearly acts like a physical substance as well as an emotion.[56] Over time, the word *cholos* lost most of its physical signification and *cholê* became the standard word for bile. But an association remains between the bitterness of anger and the bitterness of bile. Although it was only in medieval times that the theory of the four humors associated with four personality types was fully developed, healers in the fifth century had already associated the movement of bile with disease and passion. Medea's anger, her high emotions, are presented in terms of a disease which she herself is guiding and controlling.[57] At the same time, the Nurse (and Medea) insists that Jason's actions have caused 'the dearest things' to be 'sick' (νοσεῖ τὰ φίλτατα, 16), *for* (γὰρ, 17) he has betrayed Medea and his children.[58]

---

[55] For organs, cf. most notoriously, the womb: see Lefkowitz (1981) with the chapter entitled, 'The Wandering Womb' and King (1998) 214–220. For the importance of moving fluids in disease, see Padel (1992) 81–88.

[56] See especially *Iliad* 1.189–192. Smith (1966) discusses the use of the word in Homer, showing how the epic use anticipates the portrait of bile in the Hippocratic Corpus. For the history of the word χόλος/χόλη, see Chantraine (1968/1988), vol. 2, 1267–1268; for the semantics of *cholos*, see Padel (1992) 23–24.

[57] On Medea's control of the situation (and its implication for our understanding of gender roles in the play and in Attic society), see Foley (2001) 257–262, with additional bibliography given on 261 n. 65. Foley stresses the gradual emergence of Medea's 'masculine' sense of agency, 'as she shrugs off the mask of subservience' (261) worn at the beginning of the play; she argues that her masculine heroic side is hinted at early in the play, but remains disguised by Medea's own rhetoric.

[58] Jason's name (which should mean 'healer') deserves some comment. Mackie (2001) argues that Jason had been a healing figure in the earliest mythic traditions and points to indications of this tradition in Pindar, *Pythian* 4 (104–115, 156–157, 270–271). Euripides makes no obvious puns (at least that I can find) on Jason's name even as he uses medical imagery throughout the play. However, it seems possible that he deliberately undercuts any potential claims of Jason to be a healer (especially in contrast to Medea), as he suggests that Jason overestimates his own ability to solve problems. Thus, here at 16–17, Jason has created an unhealthy situation; at 548–567, he argues that he has planned well, but the play shows he has not (see further discussion in the text below). Finally, at 926, he tells Medea that he will set things right (εὖ ... ἐγὼ θήσω) for Medea and the children in Corinth, but Medea rejects his assistance; Jason's expression is not uncommon, but we do see it used in *Hippolytus* in the struggle between Phaedra and the Nurse to decide who will 'set things right' for Phaedra (cf. 521, 709, both discussed above in my analysis of *Hippolytus*). Hence, it may be that Euripides is using the expression to indicate here, as elsewhere in the play, that Jason and Medea are like

The Nurse thus is able render a diagnosis, but her prognosis for the situation is unusual, in that it concerns not Medea as patient, but rather Medea as agent: the Nurse is concerned for the welfare of the children. Moreover, although the Nurse may be able to diagnose and to suggest a possible prognosis, she cannot prescribe. The Nurse feels powerless to help Medea; she has no remedy to offer—not even the supposedly healing power of music (190–204)—and can only try to keep the children away from their mother's 'bull-like glance' (92).[59] It is rather Medea who has the power of action; it she who 'moves her anger' and who seems to have the power to heal herself.

Medical language appears early on in the play, both in the Nurse's speech and in Medea's, as, for example, when she wishes that Jason and his new bride may be 'gnawed away' (διακναιομένους, 164) together with their house. *Diaknaiô* is a word confined in fifth-century prose to medical texts where it describes laceration, both internal and external;[60] it occurs elsewhere only in drama, and even then remains fairly rare.[61] The physical semantics of this word should not be ignored in our reading here: the daughter of Creon will be lacerated in a very physical way indeed.

When Medea actually appears on stage, she hardly cuts the figure of a woman rendered sick and prostrate by her husband's betrayal. Her speech to the chorus of Corinthian women shows her to be very much in control, for all her talk of the powerlessness of women.[62] In contrast to other 'sick' characters such as Heracles, Orestes, and Phaedra, Medea feels no need to hide in shame—the shame belongs to Jason and not to her. Instead she is determined to show herself and to reveal her true inner self, her *splanchnon* (220).[63] Her situation as foreigner and her

---

healers with two competing visions of how to solve a problem (in this case, exile)—and Jason is proved incompetent in comparison with the extremely capable Medea.

[59] The Nurse in *Medea* is not, however, a good example of an incompetent healer, precisely because she makes no attempt to heal her 'patient'—and, indeed, she recognizes her inability to help Medea.

[60] *Morb.* 1.13; *Morb. Mul.* 1.64, 66; *Morb. Mul.* 2.113, 120, 121.

[61] The word appears at Aesch. *Ag.* 65, *PV* 94, 451; Eur. *Alc.* 109, *Heraclid.* 296, *El.*1307, *IA* 27, *Cyc.* 486, and here at *Med.* 164; Ar. *Pax* 251, *Ran.* 1128, *Eccl.* 957, fr. 63. 2 Kock.

[62] Mastronarde stresses the contrast between the weak Medea we expect to see given the opening scenes and the powerful Medea who actually appears (commentary, p. 205).

[63] In emphasizing the use of the word *splanchnon* here, I am indebted to the lengthy discussion of the role of *splanchna* in Greek thought by Padel (1992), esp. 13–18; the author analyzes the function of *splanchna* in ritual and the use of the term in poetry.

reputation for *authadeia* (wilfulness, self-reliance) have subjected her to injudicious hatred and fear (222–224). Yet this is not her true nature, she argues to the women of Corinth: she is a woman, just as they are, whose primary task is childbirth. People who judge from a position of ignorance (ἀμαθίας ὕπο, 224), before they have examined closely the *splanchna* of an individual—these people are to be criticized. This emphasis on learning and on inquiry into the inner self places Medea into the category of sophistic thinkers. Moreover, she aims to discover some way and device (ἤν μοι πόρος τις μηχανή τ᾽ ἐξευρεθῇ) to pay back her husband for his poor treatment of her (260–261). However, for all her efforts to be transparent here, even to the extent of announcing her vengeful, murderous intentions, she soon turns to the use of deceitful ways, of 'soft' words (316), in her attempt to convince Creon to let her stay in Corinth for only one more day. Here she claims that she is not 'exceedingly clever' (ἄγαν σοφή, 305), but in fact she is, and Creon has every reason to fear her. He recognizes her tactics and wants no part of any soft treatment that he knows he will regret later (290–291). Indeed he is right to fear that she will wreak some 'incurable evil' (ἀνήκεστον κακόν, 283) on his daughter. Nevertheless, Medea manages to persuade him with her words:[64] Creon accedes to her request for one more day in Corinth, but this proves to be all she needs to wreak her vengeance.

In her speech after Creon's exit, Medea first exults in her ability to deceive and then turns to consider various prescriptions for vengeance. She finally decides upon the method in which she is 'especially wise': the use of *pharmaka* (384–385). She urges herself to use all her skill: ἀλλ᾽ εἶα φείδου μηδὲν ὧν ἐπίστασαι, / Μήδεια, βουλεύουσα καὶ τεχνωμένη (401–402: 'but come, spare nothing of what you know, Medea, in plotting and contriving'). At the end of her speech, she returns to her earlier attempts to ally her feelings and actions with those of women in general:

> ἐπίστασαι δέ· πρὸς δὲ καὶ πεφύκαμεν
> γυναῖκες. ἐς μὲν ἔσθλ᾽ ἀμηχανώταται,
> κακῶν δὲ πάντων τέκτονες σοφώταται.   (407–409)

---

[64] Medea's ability to persuade is surely good evidence for Gorgias' argument in the *Encomium of Helen* (DK 82 B11) regarding the overwhelming power of the *logos* (which, he claims, acts like a drug).

But you understand: we are born
women, most incapable of noble things,
but the cleverest fashioners of evils.

Women are the cleverest crafters of evils, she asserts, but the play has
already begun to show how very extraordinary Medea is. Although
her reference to Hecate as her special protector (395–397) plays up the
folk-lore element of 'Medea as witch,' the emphasis on *technê*, *boulêmata*,
sophia and *pharmaka* here and elsewhere in the play all serve to reinforce
the image of Medea as a skillful and sophisticated healer gone wrong, a
healer who has set out to harm rather than to help.[65]

The great agôn between Jason and Medea extends the use of medical ideas in describing the relationship between the two. Medea defines
Jason's act of coming to see her in her distress as an act of shamelessness, 'the greatest of all diseases among humankind' (471). She proceeds
to speak to him abusively in order to 'relieve' her soul and to give him
pain (473–474). In her speech, she stresses first all her previous actions
on Jason's behalf, then descries his broken oaths and lastly points out
her lack of other resources or places of refuge. Yet she begins and ends
this central portion of her rhesis with the words 'I saved you,' (ἔσωσά σε
at both 476, 515), words that stress her resourcefulness, her power and
her ability. Moreover, we should bear in mind that Medea's methods of
saving Jason always involve physical harm to others: the killing of the
fleece-guarding dragon (a killing to which she here lays claim [482]),
the killing of her brother (acknowledged elsewhere in the play [167])
and the killing of Pelias (486). According to other sources for the story,
the deaths of brother Absyrtus and king Pelias involved extreme bodily dislocation—they were both cut up into little bits. Medea's methods
thus involve breaking bodies apart, rather than making them whole.
Finally, Medea ends her speech by praying for a stamp of character on
the exterior of the body which would act as a clear proof of a person's
true nature, a means by which one might 'see through' (διειδέναι, 518)
a bad person. Earlier in the play, it was she who had insisted on the
importance of examining the *splanchna* of human beings before judging
them; here, however, she acknowledges the real difficulty of examining
the human interior because of the opacity of the human body.[66]

---

[65] On the witch element in the Euripides play, see the summary in Mastronarde,
24–26; see also Knox (1977), who argues that Euripides has deliberately distanced his
Medea from the sorceress in other versions of the myth (see esp. 306–309).

[66] Cf. the discussion above (p. 35) of the healer's use of external signs to judge

Jason's reply indicates that Medea's efforts to cause him pain with her speech have had some effect: he begins by saying at 524–525 that he must try to 'outrun the pain induced by your tongue (γλωσσαλγία).' The speech reveals Jason as a man who has been trained in sophistic debating techniques, but is not very good at them. He begins by attributing his success to the compelling influence of the goddess Aphrodite on Medea; while admitting the cleverness of Medea's mind, he insists that responsibility for his safety rests ultimately with the gods (526–531). Furthermore, his position is due not to her *technê*, but rather to *tychê*, impersonal chance or fortune (544).[67] Even as he rejects the value of Medea's technical skills, Jason tries to beat Medea at her own game by showing that he is clever, too. He argues at 548–549, that he is both *sophos* (clever) and *sôphrôn* (prudent) and moreover that he has 'discovered a discovery' (553) which would rid him of his unmanageable troubles (συμφορὰς ἀμηχάνους, 552). His marriage is then explained as a way to help the family escape poverty—'surely I have not planned poorly?' he asks (567). Thus, Jason asserts the power of the gods, of *tychê*, and of his own clever reasoning. Unfortunately for Jason, the only divine-like figure to appear in this play is Medea herself;[68] likewise, Jason has underestimated the power of Medea's *technê* and overestimated his own. He has not been so *sophos* after all.

Medea herself stresses not her wildness but rather the cleverness (*sophia*) and self-reliance (*authadeia*) for which she is well-known (*sophia*: 285, 303, 384–385, 409, 539, 677; *authadeia*: 104, 223, 621, 1028).[69] She insists on human responsibility and human capacity for action; she resists Jason's efforts to make divine forces responsible for their history. She contains within her own body all the elements necessary to account for her actions: *thumos, megalosplanchnia* (large inner organs), *kardia* (heart), *cholos, sophia, authadeia, thasos* (boldness), *agrion êthos* (savage character).[70] The combination of these qualities has served to help

---

interior conditions. The difficulty of judging human character from exterior signs is also a common topos in tragedy; cf., e.g., *Hipp.* 925–927; *Her.* 655–672; *El.* 367–372.

[67] We might recall that the author of *The Art* maintains heatedly that medicine heals not by *tychê*, but by *technê* (cf. esp. 4–7); the ferocity of his argument suggests that, like Jason, not everyone in the fifth century was convinced of the reliability of *technê*.

[68] This is especially clear at the end of the play, when she appears as her own *dea ex machina* in the chariot (probably drawn by serpents: cf. Mastronarde *ad* 1317) supplied to her by her grandfather Helius.

[69] Medea also plays down her *sophia* in the scene with Creon in order to get what she wants (cf. 409).

[70] For *megalosplanchnia*, see 109–110, where the Nurse describes her as a μεγαλόσπλαγ-

Jason in the past and will serve to hurt him now. Jason's betrayal of his oath to her through his marriage to another undermines her stable position in Greek society.

Peaceful relations between husband and wife meant safety (μεγίστη ... σωτηρία), said the Nurse in the prologue, but now everything is inimical and the dearest things are sick (14–16). Yet, in the early stages of the play, the Nurse indicates that disaster can still be averted. She explains that Medea's sickness has not yet reached its height, but is only in its beginning stages (ἐν ἀρχῇ πῆμα κοὐδέπω μεσοῖ, 60). Nevertheless it is a powerful force, so strong that the Nurse expresses her fears of destruction: 'we shall indeed be destroyed if we add a new evil to the old one before it is drained off' (ἀπωλόμεσθ' ἄρ', εἰ κακὸν προσοίσομεν / νέον παλαιῷ, πρὶν τόδ' ἐξηντληκέναι, 78–79).[71] An additional round of evils could send Medea off on a very destructive path—and it does. Creon's decision to banish her completely disrupts her tenuous balance. Medea's pain cannot be 'drained off.' Moreover, the total of her sickness cannot be dissipated; it can only be transferred. The Nurse fears that Medea will not cease from her anger until she attacks someone: οὐδὲ παύσεται χόλου, σάφ' οἶδα, πρὶν κατασκῆψαί τινι (93–94).[72] Later in the play, Medea speaks of 'lightening her soul' (κουφισθήσομαι ψυχήν, 473–474). *Kouphizô* is commonly used by medical writers to describe alleviation of symptoms.[73] As we have seen, Medea alleviates her own pain by abusing Jason verbally and making him feel pain. Little wonder that Jason speaks of trying to escape from her *glôssalgia*, the pain induced by her tongue (524–525). At the end of the play, Medea in triumph explains the reasoning behind her terrible deeds: τῆς σῆς γὰρ ὡς χρῆν καρδίας ἀνθηψάμην (1360: 'for I have struck your heart in return, as was necessary'). When Jason protests that she shares in this pain (1361), she replies σάφ' ἴσθι· λύει δ' ἄλγος ἢν σὺ μὴ 'γγελᾷς (1362:

χνος δυσκατάπαυστος ψυχή (a proposed emendation is μελανόσπλαγχνος); *agrion êthos* occurs at 103. Other attributes have been cited above in the text. It has been proposed that the reference to *megalo-* (*melano-*) *splanchnia* characterizes Medea as a melancholic, given to depressive and angry tendencies; lines 659 and 691 are cited in support. See Guardasole (2000) 235–238.

[71] Cf. the five instances of ἀντλέω ('drain') in *Nat. Puer.* 25.

[72] For use of the verb κατασκήπτω in the Hippocratic Corpus, see *Epid.* 3.8, where it describes a disease attacking the body. It occurs more often in medical texts of the Hellenistic and Roman periods.

[73] See the discussion of Van Brock (1961) 211–212 and for this play, see Mastronarde *ad loc.*

'know well: it dissolves/relieves my pain if you do not laugh').[74] Thus, using the language of medicine to indicate very physical transactions, the play represents a shifting of a painful disease from one person to another, not a dissolution of the illness itself. Indeed, during this last exchange with Jason, Medea cries, ὦ παῖδες, ὡς ὤλεσθε πατρῴᾳ νόσῳ (1364: 'o children, how you have been destroyed by your father's disease'). Jason has now become diseased, helplessly looking up at Medea above him, replacing the image of the sick Medea at the beginning of the play, lying prone, her face fixed on the ground, paradoxically similar to a hard rock or a fluid wave as she resists the advice of well-wishers. In our final view of her, Medea is almost literally relieved of the weight of her troubles as she ascends to the sky in a sort of apotheosis. She has claimed to be heavy (*bareia*) against her enemies (809); now, at the end of the play, by burdening them, she has lightened both her soul and her body.

In the scenes that follow the agon between Medea and Jason, we watch the development and execution of Medea's plans. To achieve her ends, Medea avails herself of two elements which epitomize the fifth-century definition of human beings and which distinguish them from animals: language and *technê*.[75] She decides upon two strategies, the use of 'soft words' and the use of *pharmaka*, her particular specialty. Yet, Medea's use of her human skills is distinguished from realm of human norms as well. Medea claims to be *sophos*, but, significantly, she never claims to be *sôphrôn* except when she is lying to achieve her nefarious ends (cf. 884–885). The chorus praises *sôphrosynê* as the finest gift of the gods (636), but it does not reject Medea despite her rather obvious lack of this quality. For Medea is both ineluctable and attractive, like Aphrodite/Kypris, whose power is now wonderful, now inconvenient. Just as Aphrodite smears her love-inducing arrows with desire (χρυσέων τόξων … / ἱμέρῳ χρίσασ᾽ ἄφυκτον οἰστόν, 633–635), Medea gives gifts smeared with *pharmaka* (τοιοῖσδε χρίσω φαρμάκοις δωρήματα, 789), gifts too lovely to be refused. Divine power is incontestable and not to be contested. Sophia and Eros, which the chorus praises as a combination

---

[74] Over 200 uses of the verb λύω appear in the Hippocratic Corpus. See Maloney and Frohn (1984) v. III, 2493–2497. It is frequently used to express the 'resolution' of a disease: thus, common usages include λύει τὸ νόσημα (*Aph.* 2.21; 4.57, 58; *Coac.* 448; *Judic.* 61); λύει τὴν ὀδύνην (*Reg. Acut.* 5, 7; *Epid.* 2.26; *Epid.* 4.1.40; *Morb. Mul.* 2.128); λύει τὸ ἄλγος/ τάς ἀλγηδόνας (*Reg. Acut.* 7; *Aph.* 4.11; 5.25; *Coac.* 539, 542; *Pror.* 1.145).

[75] Heinimann (1961: 108 with notes 16 and 17) discusses the fifth-century view that *technê* was an important element in the distinction between humans and animals.

of traits exemplified by the Athenians, are also combined in Medea, but the play shows the destructive power of these forces in human life when they are not also tempered by a third important element, *sôphrosynê*. To be *sôphrôn* is to know one's human limitations, to remain within the appropriate boundaries of the human mind; the gods, by contrast, are not bound by such respect for limitations. Once established in Greece, Medea is willing to accept the rules thrust upon her by Greek society, as long as everyone in that society follows those rules. But when Jason breaks his oath of loyalty to her, she recognizes the fragility of those rules, and she refuses to submit to Greek norms for human conduct any longer. Shared submission to the laws of society results in harmony, but excesses by one group or the disregard of conventions can lead to the breakdown of the entire system. Perhaps not surprisingly given the contemporary debates over the whether *physis* (nature) or *nomos* (law or custom) predominates in the affairs of humankind, the play, which on the one hand seems to emphasize issues of *physis* (such as the particular nature of women as opposed to men), at the same time pushes the issue of *nomos* very hard.[76]

The gruesome tale of the death of Creon's daughter and of Creon himself, victims of Medea's *technê* so angrily applied, is the precursor to the ultimate act of terror, the mother's killing of her children. Through these increasingly horrific acts, Medea is removed from the realm of the human, based as it seems to be on a shared set of assumptions and limitations; indeed, at the end of the play, Jason rejects her human identity entirely, defining her instead as a lioness wilder than the monster Scylla (1342–1343). But if she is an animal, she is one with incredible power over him; if she is an animal, then the traditional hierarchy of human over animal has been reversed; the laws of nature have been overturned, the rivers flow backwards just as they have been described in the chorus' song (410). Through her *technê*, Medea has achieved an inversion of *physis*; she has been spurred to do so by Jason's inversion of *nomos*.

The *Medea* shows the danger of *technê* and *sophia* misapplied, or applied in the absence of restraint. Medea is determined to heal herself by destroying others; she has no interest in the well being of 'patients'

---

[76] The *nomos-physis* debate turns up in just about every genre of Greek literature in the fifth century, including the Hippocratic Corpus (most obviously in *Airs, Waters, Places*; cf. esp. 14 and 24). For scholarly discussion, see Heinimann (1945) and Kerferd (1981) ch. 10.

other than herself—and her children, whom she kills, she claims, so that they will not suffer (1060–1061).[77] Medea is very good at what she does, and she accomplishes exactly what she sets out to do. Of course, this reading of the play has been quite unsympathetic to Medea. Certainly Medea's status as woman, barbarian and abandoned wife places her in a position of weakness, and the play sets forth complex motivations for her behavior. Moreover, her decision to kill her children, though horrific, is based on a set of ethical principles endorsed in traditional Greek thought, as Christopher Gill has shown.[78] Medea knows that she will suffer from her own actions, but she believes that by sharing her pain with Jason, she will lessen her own. Once again, we see the attitude of *Breaths'* author reconfigured: the healer suffers along with the patient, but this time the healer has caused the pain.

Thus far, we have seen images of healers allied with characters who are either low status or wildly 'other.' Now let us turn to examine some characters who are represented as powerful by virtue of their position in society but are unable to exercise their power successfully. These characters, not surprisingly male, seem to have some grasp of medical *technê* but are nonetheless limited in their ability to practice it, either by their own choice or by circumstances beyond their control. The first type is represented by Menelaus in *Orestes*, the second by several figures in Sophocles: Oedipus in *Oedipus Tyrannus*, Philoctetes, Aias. Although *Orestes*, a play in which disease themes and images are manifold, will receive fuller treatment in Part II of this study, it will be useful to focus on the character of Menelaus in the context currently under discussion. For Menelaus, as we will see, conducts his initial visit with his stricken nephew in many ways like a medical interview;[79] however, he concludes that the case is a hopeless one and decides to retire from the scene. By contrast, Oedipus, Philoctetes and Aias are central to their own cases and remain firm in their determination to handle the disease under their care without flinching. Their chosen course of action—even if productive of truth—nonetheless has potentially or actually destructive consequences. Thus, these characters each to some extent build upon

---

[77] The authenticity of these lines, which comprise part of a much disputed portion of Medea's speech at 1019–1080, is contested. Mastronarde accepts them as genuine, Diggle and Kovacs do not. For a useful overview of the problem, see the Appendix in Mastronarde's commentary on the play (pp. 388–393).

[78] Gill (1996a) 154–174.

[79] Willink *ad* 385–447 describes Menelaus' attitude as 'doctor-like.'

the model of the knowledgeable healer who cannot heal himself so eloquently established in *Prometheus Bound*. The cases of Philoctetes and Aias mirror that of Prometheus closely, in that these two characters both suffer from disease themselves: Philoctetes cannot ultimately heal his disease himself and thus must rely in the end on the resources of the society that had earlier spurned him; Aias manages to recover from madness but not from its consequences, and he finds the only remedy for his situation to be death itself. Oedipus sets out to heal the plague afflicting his fellow citizens, but he himself is ultimately revealed to be the source of the disease.

The influence of medical ideas on Sophocles' portrait of Oedipus in *Oedipus Tyrannus* has been incisively analyzed by Bernard Knox. Knox has demonstrated the ways in which Oedipus is assimilated to a healer as he seeks a cure for the plague that ails the city.[80] In the opening scenes, Oedipus is shown at least one step ahead of his 'patients' on several counts. Yet Oedipus, for all his intelligence, is proven tragically ignorant. It is his ignorance of the past and even of the present that ultimately renders him patient rather than healer. As noted earlier, the opening section of the treatise *Prognostic* stresses that the good healer (like successful prophets and poets) must know past, present and future.[81] Oedipus, despite all his efforts on behalf of the city, despite his cleverness, does not know the truth of the past or of the present; thus, he cannot successfully predict the outcome of the case, try as he might. However, Sophocles' presentation of Oedipus as a man of science should not be read as a thorough condemnation of human intellectual abilities. Rather, Oedipus should be understood as representative of the potential dangers and ultimate limitations of the pursuit of knowledge and authority. Oedipus, after all, does not fail to discover the truth, but—like many healers in the late fifth century— he cannot with any surety effect a cure, either of his own suffering or of the suffering of others.[82] Within the space and time of the play,

---

[80] Knox (1957) 139–147. Knox has not persuaded everyone—Kamerbeek admires his argument, but resists it in the details; see Kamerbeek's commentary on the *OT*, pp. 26–27.

[81] Cf. above pp. 30–31 with note 30.

[82] Sophocles perhaps gestures to the healers' claim, expressed in *Breaths* 1, to suffer more than the patient, in that they participate in more than their own suffering. Oedipus suffers doubly in that he is both healer and patient, dealing with an unimaginably terrible 'disease.'

it is never explicitly said that the plague (which, it has been noticed, receives less and less attention as the play continues) is cured. The oracle reported by Creon states that the person responsible for the death of Laius must be removed (in some way) from Thebes. However, at the end of the play, when Oedipus asks to be removed from the land as quickly as possible (1436), Creon hesitates—and Oedipus remains in Thebes, at least until another play can come and get him out. Moreover, Creon's stubborn insistence that he cannot expel Oedipus until he gets further instructions from the god (1438–1439, 1442–1443) seems rather suspect to me: after all, according to Creon himself, the earlier oracle he had obtained from Delphi had spoken clearly (ἐμφανῶς, 96) enough as to what was required. Throughout the play, despite the clarity of the oracle emphasized by Creon in his report, the answer to the question regarding the exact nature of the cure has remained ambiguous: is it to be exile or death? Creon's unwillingness to expel Oedipus—which is emphasized by the poet—may indicate that Creon considers death, not exile, to be the appropriate remedy. Nevertheless, even while including all these discussions about the need for remedy, Sophocles seems deliberately to avoid resolution as to the specific fates of Oedipus and the population of Thebes. The possibility that Oedipus may have provided the cure to the plague, but that the cure will be set aside for political gain on the part of Creon lies open. The determination of Oedipus to heal his city through decisive action is—perhaps—thwarted by the caution of Creon.

e. Orestes: *No heroic measures*

If Oedipus is quick to act and sure of his own abilities, the same can hardly be said for the doctor figure in *Orestes*. The encounter between Orestes and Menelaus, as commentators have pointed out, is replete with language and gestures also prominent in the realm of Hippocratic medicine. Menelaus plays the role of doctor, Orestes, that of patient. But commentators have failed to note, I believe, how curiously doctor and patient behave. The patient begins by claiming that his body is already destroyed, and that only his name remains; however, it later becomes clear that the patient still hopes for a complete recovery—with the aid of the doctor. It is the patient, Orestes, who provides a sophisticated self-diagnosis of *synesis*, 'self-awareness' or 'conscience' (ἡ σύνεσις, ὅτι σύνοιδα δείν' εἰργασμένος, 396: 'self-awareness, that I am aware that I have done terrible things')[83]—too sophisticated in fact for the doctor Menelaus to understand. Moreover, it is the patient who suggests a remedy and the doctor who (after the interruption of Tyndareus at least) hesitates to act on behalf of the patient. On the other hand, the doctor does manage to isolate the two-fold nature of the threats against his patient. His questions divide Orestes' difficulties into two categories, those for which divine powers are evidently responsible and those which derive from human society. Significantly, Orestes' initial self-diagnosis of *synesis* as the cause of his *nosos* can account for all his difficulties. But his awareness that he has done terrible things is not a disease which anyone but Orestes himself could treat.

When Menelaus arrives at the palace in Argos where Orestes lies sick, he has been long awaited by Orestes and Electra as their only hope of avoiding death (52–53; 67–70). But his opening speech is not encouraging: he condemns the killing of Clytemnestra as an 'unholy murder' (ἀνόσιον φόνον, 374), even though he is distressed at the murder of Agamemnon.[84] He seeks his nephew, not knowing what he will look like after all these years (375–379). In the ensuing lines, Orestes identifies himself and makes a plea for Menelaus' help. As the two begin their conversation, several odd features characterize the medical and sophistic language that peppers the exchange. First, it is Orestes who defines Menelaus' role as a healer and at the same time, it is Orestes who not only describes and diagnoses his own disease, but also suggests a cure. Thus, Orestes exclaims to his uncle that he has arrived ἐς καιρόν ('at just the right time,' 384) to save him. The notion of *kairos* is essential in the Hippocratic Corpus.[85] For the Hippocratics, disease may be localized, but it is not caused by germs or viruses; rather, it is a process, involving a battle between different forces in the body.[86]

---

[83] There is an extensive literature on this term and its significance for the play: in particular, see Rodgers (1969), Porter (1994) 298–313, Garzya (1997), Guardasole (2000) 211–219.

[84] If we accept (with Degani, Reeve and Willink) Dindorf's deletion of 361, then Menelaus did not hear about Clytemnestra's role in the murder of Agamemnon until his return to Argos, when he also learned of the murder of Clytemnestra. But although Dindorf's arguments may be persuasive, Menelaus' quickly formed negative verdict on his nephew's actions—judged at least in the Homeric and Aeschylean versions of the story to be the necessary, even if horrific, response to Clytemnestra's deeds—is nonetheless striking. For discussion of Dindorf's deletion and responses to it, see Willink *ad loc*.

[85] See Jouanna (1999) 344.

[86] On the Hippocratic notion of disease as process, see Grmek (1989) 293; for the

Such forces may receive reinforcements from external substances or be offset by counter measures performed by the healer, but timing is a critical part of the process. The experienced healer knows that different diseases respond to intervention at different times and he must learn to discern the appropriate time to treat each disease. Indeed, the author of *On the Sacred Disease* asserts that the good healer could heal any disease if he understands the principles of regimen and 'if he could distinguish the right times for applying [the remedies]' (εἰ τοὺς καιροὺς διαγινώσκοι τῶν συμφερόντων, 18.6). Orestes is actually sick, as the opening scene with Electra makes clear, and at the same time the whole situation is sick, as the disease imagery of the play underscores throughout. His case demands treatment now—according to the patient. The words of his uncle, however, are hardly encouraging: he takes one look at Orestes and places him already in the category of the dead (τίνα δέδορκα νερτέρων;, 385: 'which of the dead do I see?'). As Orestes explains that he may look awful, but he is still alive, Menelaus continues to emphasize the extent of Orestes' physical deterioration (387, 389, 391). Even Orestes admits that he does not have much life left in him, agreeing that his body is gone, but protesting that his name still remains (390).

Menelaus' attitude towards Orestes is more shocked than sympathetic, but Orestes presses on, determined to enlist Menelaus in his struggle. After reviewing the condition of Orestes' body, the two men turn to a discussion of the cause and nature of his disease. The murder of Clytemnestra clearly plays a part in it, but the conversation seeks to find a more specific diagnosis. Again, for all that Orestes seeks help from Menelaus, Menelaus is depicted as hardly knowledgeable or skilled. After Menelaus examines Orestes' external *amorphia* (disfigurement, 391), he does not then proceed to diagnose the patient but instead asks the patient to diagnose himself: τίς σ᾿ ἀπόλλυσιν νόσος; (395: 'What disease is destroying you?'). Then begins a discussion of internal diseases or internal factors causing disease. When Orestes names *synesis* as his disease at 396, admitting that he has done 'terrible things,'[87] Menelaus fails to understand and asks for a clearer explanation (397).

importance of war, politics and competition in Greek ideas of disease, see Vegetti (1983) and Jouanna (1999) 141.

[87] The Greek word is *deina*, not *kaka* or *adika*; it has the sense of 'awesome' or 'amazing,' and does not have the clear moral import that *kaka* or *adika* would have. Euripides leaves Orestes' attitude towards the murder of his mother ambiguous throughout the play; sometimes, Orestes justifies his actions, sometimes, he expresses regret and horror over what he has done.

Orestes then proceeds to give a more customary set of causal factors, grief and madness.[88] He first names *lypê* (grief) as that which is destroying him (398), and here Menelaus responds for the first and only time with a note of optimism: δείνη γὰρ ἡ θεός, ἀλλ᾽ ὅμως ἰάσιμος (399: 'terrible is the goddess, but nonetheless subject to cure'). This optimism is soon dimmed, however, as Orestes goes on to add that he also suffers from madness (400). Menelaus asks for details about the madness: when did it begin, was he at home or outside when it happened, has anyone been helping Orestes through it, what are the details of his insane visions (401–407)? But when Orestes at 412 bemoans his suffering, Menelaus gives us yet another hint that things are not going to go well for Orestes in this matter: instead of offering a cure or reassurance, he responds that those who do terrible things suffer terribly in turn (413). Indeed, in the next line it is Orestes who suggests that there is a cure for what ails him—not death, against which Menelaus counsels— but the help of Apollo. Menelaus again responds pessimistically: Apollo has not come yet, but the Furies have arrived quickly (419–423). It is reiterated that this is the sixth day of Orestes' illness (422; cf. 39). The precision of this information may have medical connotations as well as ritual ones, for many Greek rationalist healers were firm believers in the doctrine of 'critical days,' days on which a disease reached a turning point and would either become worse or better. Different diseases had different critical days, so it was important to get a complete picture of the patient's symptoms and attempt to pinpoint the nature of the disease in order to be able to discern the critical days in question. Different treatises employ different systems of establishing critical days and may also suggest that individual diseases operate with their own particular patterns. Some Hippocratic treatises that address the issue establish odd days as critical days, but most writers actually tend to stress both odd and even days, with the fourth, seventh and fourteenth regularly cited as likely.[89] According to *Epidemics* 1 and 3, both odd and even days can be critical, and in fact, this treatise seems particularly concerned to establish that there are medical periods that involve even days—as Volker Langholf has suggested, the author of this group of *Epidemics* may be trying to show a correlation between paroxysms and

---

[88] Willink *ad* 396 points to the paradox of Orestes suffering from *synesis* and *mania* at the same time.

[89] Cf. in particular, *Reg. Acut.* 4, *Coac.* 147–148, *Dieb. Judic.* 11, *Prog.* 20.

crises on even days.[90] It seems possible that, given the medical language
that pervades the scene, Menelaus' enquiry into the length of Orestes'
illness may have medical implications as well.[91] If this is a critical day,
we may expect Orestes to get significantly better or worse; furthermore,
we may also expect some decisive action from the 'doctor' Menelaus.
However, yet again, Menelaus renders no judgment but continues his
assessment of Orestes' situation. Now he begins to ask about Orestes'
allies in the struggle. Orestes despairingly admits he has none, that his
prospects in the city look grim. Death by stoning awaits him, no escape
routes are open.

At last, Menelaus is prepared to give his diagnosis—and, surely, his
prognosis: ὦ μέλεος, ἥκεις συμφορᾶς ἐς τοὔσχατον (447: 'o wretched one,
you have come to the final point of disaster'). Menelaus apparently has
no help to offer, no remedy to provide.[92] The situation is desperate.
Orestes, however, is not ready to let his uncle off the hook so easily.
He points out that in fact it is Menelaus who is his source of refuge
from the evils that beset him (448). Before the two can discuss this
matter further, however, they are interrupted by the arrival of Tyndareus, whose furious criticism of Orestes' actions seems to weaken
any inclination that Menelaus may have to help his nephew enthusi-
astically. After Tyndareus leaves, Menelaus' response to Orestes' pleas
is to preach caution (*eulabeia*) and to wait for the right time (*kairos*).[93]
Clearly, Menelaus and Orestes disagree as to the timing and the kind
of intervention necessary. As we will see in greater detail in Part II of
this study, the whole question of intervention is fraught with difficulties
for the medical writers; intervention may hurt the patient more than
help, and damage to the patient is not only unfortunate in itself, but
potentially harmful to the healer's reputation as well. If Orestes' case is

---

[90] Langholf (1990) 113–118 and on the concept of critical days more generally, 79–
118. See also Jouanna (1999) 338–340.

[91] It may even be possible that Euripides' use of the six day period indicates a
general public awareness of the particular debate over the relationship of odd and even
to critical days that appears in *Epidemics* 1 and 3 (these treatises date to around 410 B.C.,
according to Deichgräber [1933] 16).

[92] Porter (1994: 70–71) maintains that Menelaus is sympathetic to Orestes' situation
and that only the violent threats of Tyndareus cause him to change his mind. However,
it seems to me that the expressions of sympathy, appropriate as they may be to his
'doctor' role, nevertheless do not outweigh the strong impression he gives that he can
do nothing to help Orestes; this attitude is then only strengthened by the words of
Tyndareus in the agon.

[93] See especially 699.

truly desperate, then attempting to intervene is problematic. Menelaus' solution may make some medical sense, but it is clearly directed also at preserving his own self-interest and reputation.[94] For Menelaus does not refuse to help Orestes outright; instead, he suggests some gentle, indirect approaches—the use of 'soft words,' the attempt to win over Tyndareus. He will try to save Orestes with *sophia*, not *bia* (force). However, as we have seen, Menelaus is not portrayed as particularly *sophos*. It seems likely that his attempts will fail. In the world of Euripides' *Orestes*, persuasion always fails; violence appears to be the only kind of solution, yet even violence provides no way out. The problem of 'no way out' (*aporia*), stressed in the opening scenes of the play (70, 232, 315), rules the day—until the miracle of divine intervention appears to settle matters.

Technê, so often celebrated in the fifth century as one of the special qualities that makes human beings distinctive, is fundamental to the doctrines of rationalist healers. They work, so they claim, on the basis of skills that derive from a body of knowledge that they have not only learned but also can pass on to others. They practice medicine not by chance, but with consistent, reliable methods; their results are predictable. So they must be, at any rate, if medicine is to be considered a *technê*. But such optimistic claims often ran counter to the actualities of disease and treatment in the fifth century. Medicine relies on order, predictability and regularity in order to succeed. However, as Euripides is concerned to demonstrate to us—and, as the many admissions of doubt and failure found particularly in the Hippocratic *Epidemics* also reveal—order and predictability are but fleeting in the course of human life. In the next part of this study, I will investigate the theories on causation and remedy developed by the rationalist healers in their attempts to reveal the orderliness of nature and to heal their patients. Then I will explore the ways in which these theories of disease and remedial strategies are also operative in Euripidean tragedy, but this analysis will reveal that such human methods of coping with suffering and disease are often misguided or futile; even as they repeatedly try to solve problems using rational methods, the human characters of Euripidean drama are thwarted by the chaos of human existence.

---

[94] On the slipperiness of Menelaus' last speech, see Porter (1994) 71–72. He suggests that the speech is one 'of a cowardly but clever villain.' I am not sure that Menelaus can be termed clever: like Jason in *Medea*, he uses sophistic language, but his rhetoric is no match for the situation nor does it disguise the betrayal that is occurring.

PART II

FROM CAUSE TO CURE

CHAPTER THREE

THE STORY OF DISEASE

We do not come to a tragedy expecting sweetness and light. We know that suffering and loss lie at the heart of the action in the tales that tragedy has to tell. Furthermore, that suffering is subject to investigation: why do we suffer? Do we bring our troubles on ourselves or should we find fault in the largely unpredictable and undeniably powerful forces of the universe? The *Odyssey* gives, famously, an answer to these questions in the words of Zeus, who claims that humans blame the gods, when it is they who bring pains upon themselves through their own bad behavior:

> Ὦ πόποι, οἷον δή νυ θεοὺς βροτοὶ αἰτιόωνται.
> ἐξ ἡμέων γάρ φασι κάκ’ ἔμμεναι· οἱ δὲ καὶ αὐτοὶ
> σφῇσιν ἀτασθαλίῃσιν ὑπὲρ μόρον ἄλγε’ ἔχουσιν　　　　(1.32–34)

> O, how indeed mortals blame the gods,
> for from us they say that evils come: but they themselves
> have pains beyond what is allotted because of their own recklessness.

However, Zeus’ words do not suggest that suffering would not occur for mortals in the absence of these behavioral circumstances, for the suffering he addresses is suffering *hyper moron*, ‘beyond what is allotted.’ Pain is part of human existence and must be accepted as such, according to so many of our archaic sources. The wounds, plagues and diseases to which the archaic poets refer also appear in tragedy, but tragedy shows a greater interest in the specific causes and effects of disease. It is no longer enough to say that disease exists, that it is difficult to control, and that it is part of the human burden. Now we are increasingly presented with particulars: symptoms, possible causes, options for treatment. Tragic figures who are sick are likely to suffer from excess of love or madness—what we might characterize as psychological disorders. The physical symptoms manifested by men who go mad follow a fairly typical pattern,[1] but the causes are different.

---

[1] Many scholars and commentators have observed this pattern, which often includes foaming at the mouth and rolling back of the eyes. As noted in the Introduction,

Women who go mad most often do so in a Dionysiac frenzy.[2] They
are also the more likely sex to become physically sick through excessive passion. Larger groups tend to suffer from more traditional types
of disease, such as the god-sent plague in *Oedipus Tyrannus* (mentioned
specifically at 27) and the threat of widespread suffering and infertility threatened by the Furies in *Eumenides* (503–507; 780–787 = 810–817).
Occasionally cities and groups are sick with ailments which we would
not consider physical/bio-medical: the city in *Heracles* is sick with stasis
(civil strife or factionalism; cf. 34, 272–273, 542–543), the land in *Phoenissae* is sick (867), Hellas is sick along with Menelaus in *Iphigenia in Aulis*
(411). In these instances, divine causation is not obvious and certainly
not direct. Madness, erotic love, political chaos and moral weakness are
the common and rather distinctive diseases of tragedy.

The weight accorded to divine and human/natural factors in the
tragedies differs from play to play. If the audience of *Heracles* actually
sees Lyssa proclaiming *ex machina* that she will drive Heracles mad in
what seems a very clear cut instance of divine causation, the audience
of *Orestes* hears the protagonist attribute his sickness to his own sense
of guilt (396) even as he blames Apollo for his predicament and has
an on-stage battle with invisible Erinyes. The commands of Artemis
and Necessity carry less weight in *Iphigenia in Aulis* with its grumbling
army and 'sick' leaders (cf. 407–411) than in *Agamemnon*, where the
alastôr of the house of Atreus, the recurring curse (1501, 1508), suggests a
kind of inexorability to the proceedings, even if Agamemnon still must

---

the pattern is very similar to the symptoms of epilepsy, as described for example
in *On the Sacred Disease*. However, there are several important exceptions: the tragic
characters can talk during these fits of madness, whereas an epileptic cannot speak;
moreover, the tragic characters have hallucinations and delusions and they walk or
leap about—hardly exemplifiers of the 'falling sickness.' For this point, and comparison
of mad symptoms in tragedy and epileptic symptoms in the Hippocratic Corpus, see
Jouanna (1987). Epilepsy was also sometimes referred to as the 'disease of Heracles,'
a fact which has caused some scholars to align the madness suffered by Heracles in
Her. with an epileptic fit. But, arguing against this interpretation, von Staden (1992b)
points out that Euripides' description of Heracles' madness follows common patterns
of tragic *mania*, and thus a specific link between epilepsy and the madness in *Her.*
is unlikely; moreover, he reminds us that tragic *mania* shares symptoms common not
only to medical descriptions of epilepsy, but also to those of hysteria, and remarks that
although Heracles is noted for transvestism, he has never been thought to possess a
'wandering womb.'

[2] Ruth Padel has discussed the peculiar nature attributed to Greek women that
makes them particularly susceptible to inspiration or possession: see Padel (1983) and
(1992) 99–113; cf. also King (1998) 108–109.

shoulder the blame for his decision to sacrifice his daughter. Philoctetes in Sophocles' play of that name does not dwell on the possibility of divine causation for the festering wound that he received from a snake bite; his concerns are his enduring pain and his resentment of Odysseus and the other Greeks for their callous treatment of him. It is the social situation, the suffering caused by the wound and by the isolation of Philoctetes that the play emphasizes rather than any possible divine motivations in the story.[3] By contrast, Heracles, at the end of Sophocles' *Trachiniae*, comes to understand his suffering as the consequence of a long chain of events, part of the workings of his fate and beyond his personal control, even if his own actions have inevitably contributed to it.

Thus, within tragic visions of causality, there are significant variations among the reasons put forward for the mental and physical suffering of a particular individual or community. Two points are especially important for our purposes. First, tragedy allows for three types of causation: 1) direct divine intervention, 2) the so-called double determination of divine and natural factors, and 3) directly mechanistic, natural causes;[4] second, the tragedies generally seek to find meaning in suf-

---

[3] Although Philoctetes himself may not dwell on any divine causality operative in his suffering, Neoptolemus maintains at 192–200 that Philoctetes has been wounded as part of a divine plan to keep him from Troy until the time when the city is destined to fall.

[4] Euripides fr. 292 Nauck-Snell (from the lost *Bellerophon*) provides a good example of the mixed approach to disease that is so clearly present in tragedy, even if the actual nature of any particular 'mixture' remains difficult to define. In the fragment, it is maintained that the healer needs to act with circumspection when treating disease; the fragment divides diseases into two categories: πρὸς τὴν νόσον τοι καὶ τὸν ἰατρὸν χρεὼν / ἰδόντ' ἀκεῖσθαι, μὴ ἐπιτὰξ τὰ φάρμακα / διδόντ', ἐὰν μὴ ταῦτα τῇ νόσῳ πρέπῃ. / νόσοι δὲ θνητῶν αἱ μέν εἰσ' αὐθαίρετοι, / αἱ δ' ἐκ θεῶν πάρεισιν, ἀλλὰ τῷ νόμῳ / ἰώμεθ' αὐτάς. ἀλλά σοι λέξαι θέλω, / εἰ θεοί τι δρῶσιν αἰσχρόν, οὐκ εἰσὶν θεοί. ('In the case of disease it is necessary that the healer too / heal after examining, not giving drugs straightaway, / in case these not be appropriate to the disease. / Some diseases of mortals are self-inflicted, / some come from the gods, but through custom / we heal them. But I wish to say to you, / if the gods do something disgraceful, they are not gods.') One type is *authairetos* (self-chosen), the other god-sent. The two types clearly hearken back to types already present in Homer, Hesiod and Pindar. But Euripides undercuts the force of the god-sent diseases by denying that gods who 'do something base' (such as cause disease) are truly gods. (There has been some dissatisfaction with the text of the fragment; Müller [1993] suggests a lacuna starting at the middle of line 6, and Luppe [1998], picking up on Müller's argument, considers various different configurations of the final lines). Compare the sentiment expressed here on the nature of the gods with similar ideas expressed in *On the Sacred Disease* (see esp. 1.43–46 Grensemann) and cf. also above Part I, p. 31.

fering. The tragic view of disease causation differs from the medical view in that the medical writers are concerned to reject divine causation and that they try to avoid assigning meaning to illness. Medicine aspires to be non-judgmental; it does not explain the presence of disease as moral punishment or as fate. The experience of illness is not understood to be a guide for the moral evaluation of the life and character of the sufferer. I do not mean to suggest that Greek healers did not criticize patient behavior that they deemed detrimental to health—there is plenty of medical advice on healthy and unhealthy regimens which includes, for example, critiques of indolent lifestyles or excessive eating and drinking. Yet for the medical author, disease itself is impersonal, objective: it does not, in general, have meaning.[5] Once again, I must qualify this as a statement of the ideal. Theories presented in the Hippocratic Corpus reveal that assumptions about character do influence Greek medical thought. Theories of physiology and pathology are based on pre-existing views of human behavior and human differences, so that, for example, differences between male and female physiology are based on the traditional belief that women are less stable; this instability is actualized, explained by the particular physiology of women (watery, spongy, changeable). Unlike the tragedians, the medical writers of the fifth century offer no reason *why* disease should exist at all in this world—it simply does, and their job is to explain how it occurs, not why. The different components of the human body, such as blood, air, fire, bile, phlegm, water, bones, muscles and organs, interact without divine direction, and indeed often act with the passion and desire of tragic figures and the irresponsibility of Euripidean gods.

Several Hippocratic writers argue that if one can find the cause, one can find the cure. This theoretical position must have been divorced to some extent from the everyday reality that faced most healers: even if they did believe they knew the cause, whether that be excess bile, excess phlegm or some other factor, they were not very successful in curing patients suffering from infectious diseases that could not be overcome by the natural processes of the body itself. Success rates for healers in antiquity are extremely difficult to measure—and, indeed, we must also be careful about defining what 'success' might mean to the

---

[5] But see Pigeaud (1990), with his argument that the author of *On Ancient Medicine* does give meaning to disease as a bringer of culture; cf. above, Part I, pp. 47–48 with note 83.

ancients.[6] The author of *The Art* maintains that success is 'the complete removal of the sufferings of the patients' (τὸ δὴ πάμπαν ἀπαλλάσσειν τῶν νοσεόντων τοὺς καμάτους, 3.2), but surely many ancient Greeks would have had to be satisfied with less. Mirko Grmek's summaries of research in paleodemography and paleopathology indicate that Greek healers made no significant impact on the life expectancy rates of people in antiquity (although these are very difficult to calculate precisely); indeed, because of increasing population density and other social factors, life expectancy probably decreased even as Hippocratic medicine began to flourish.[7]

The stories of specific illnesses (as opposed to descriptions aimed at classifying diseases) told in the Hippocratic Corpus, above all in the *Epidemics*, take two forms: one, seen especially in the so-called *katastaseis* (general conditions) sections of the *Epidemics*, is based on characteristics of disease that mark a large and anonymous group of individuals sharing certain particulars; the other, the 'case-history,' tells the tale of a named individual.[8] Death provides the end of the story for many of these patients, both anonymous and identified. Most disease stories in the Corpus do have an end (a *krisis*, a decisive moment followed by a resolution) since most diseases addressed by the writers are acute, not chronic.[9] Likewise, the art form of the drama requires an ending, however tenuous; but drama, distinguished from the action of daily human life in so many ways, is compelled to seek resolution within certain constraints of time and space. Unlike the doctor of the *Epidemics*, for example, who might follow the sad progress of his patient's disease for days on end, the Greek tragedian had one day in which to present four plays. To be sure, death often provided an intelligible and definitive ending to the story of the individual, both in tragedy and in medicine.[10] But death was not the desired outcome—healer, patient, audience and tragic hero/heroine would in most cases

---

[6] See the cautionary remarks of King (1998) 132–157, esp. 154, and see also the work of medical anthropologists such as Kleinman (1980), who show how important cultural expectations and patterns of explanation are for the efficacy of medicine.

[7] For a review of paleopathology and paleodemography in Greece, see Grmek (1989) chapters 2 and 3; for his assessment of the impact of Hippocratic medicine, see 92.

[8] Females in the case-histories are not named but are identified by the name of their *kyrios*.

[9] Jouanna (1999) 153.

[10] On death as a particularly common strategy of closure, see Smith (1968) and Dunn (1996) 1–7.

much rather that the protagonists of both case history and drama overcome their sufferings and live happily ever after. The end of any real human life was (and remains) largely unpredictable.

Greek tragedy presents both the pathos of death experienced and the excitement of death escaped. Few characters die from 'natural' causes (i.e., old age, death in child-birth, starvation, disease) in the course of a tragedy; rather, death comes to these mythological figures in the form of murder, suicide, human sacrifice, death in battle or monstrous accident. When the threat of imminent death is avoided in tragedy, it is often accomplished through divine intervention. Indeed, critics have cited divine intervention as a hallmark of Euripidean drama, pointing to cases where the playwright seems determined to accomplish rescue through divine agency even when the human characters appear to have been solving problems quite successfully on their own.[11] The so-called romance plays *Helen* and *Iphigenia among the Taurians* are especially notorious in this regard: at the last minute, defeat is snatched from the jaws of success, trouble arises unexpectedly, and, instead of wily Greeks outwitting barbarians, we are presented with a rescuing divinity. In other plays such as *Hippolytus*, *Electra* and *Orestes*, divinities appear at the outset or act behind the scenes to control human activity. *Hippolytus* presents the vengeance of Aphrodite on the man who has spurned her cult, and it is her will that drives much of the dramatic action. In *Electra* and *Orestes*, the oracle of Apollo orders the death of Clytemnestra as punishment for her murder of Agamemnon. The *Heracles* provides a horrifying and exceptional variation on the theme of divine agency: it is only despite the terrible intervention of the gods in the middle of the play and the subsequent slaughter of his family by Heracles himself that the hero lives on, induced by the care and encouragement of human friendship. Yet this frequent appearance of divine hands at work hardly serves to forestall human attempts to fix the situation by themselves. Just as Greek healers labored on in very often futile or misguided attempts to save their patients (until Nature or Tyche came to the rescue or the patient died), so too do tragic figures attempt to resolve their problems on their own.

This discussion has served by way of a preamble to the issues of cause and cure. In this chapter, I begin with a discussion of Hippocratic attitudes on the causes of disease. I then analyze some basic

---

[11] On this particular aspect of Euripidean drama, see Burnett (1971), esp. 65–69.

principles that characterize the Greek approach to problem-solving, by investigating the most prominent therapeutic approaches in Hippo- cratic medicine. After this examination of some major issues regarding causation and remedy addressed in the medical literature, I proceed to an analysis of cause and cure in four tragedies, *Orestes, Heracles, Phoenis- sae* and *Bacchae*.

CHAPTER FOUR

CAUSES OF DISEASE IN THE HIPPOCRATIC CORPUS

Perhaps the most significant difference between the attitude towards
disease causation of the medical authorities represented in the Hippocratic Corpus and that which existed in traditional views of disease
is the issue of divine involvement. This issue has engendered a large
body of scholarship.[1] It has been noted that those few medical authors
who directly address the question of divinities do not deny the existence
of gods, but instead focus their efforts on redefining the relationship
between the gods, disease and healing. The author of *On the Sacred Disease* says that epilepsy (the *hierê nosos*) is no more divine a disease than
any other—all diseases are divine:[2]

> τὸ δὲ νόσημα τοῦτο οὐδέν τι μοι δοκεῖ θειότερον εἶναι τῶν λοιπῶν, ἀλλὰ
> φύσιν μὲν ἔχειν καὶ τὰ ἄλλα νοσήματα, ὅθεν ἕκαστα γίνεται, φύσιν δὲ τοῦτο
> καὶ πρόφασιν, καὶ ἀπὸ τοῦ αὐτοῦ θεῖον γίνεσθαι ἀφ' ὅτου καὶ τὰ ἄλλα
> πάντα.   (2.1–2 Grensemann)

> This disease seems to me in no way more divine than the rest, but to
> have natural existence in the same way as other diseases, according as
> each arises, and this one too has a natural existence and a cause, and it
> seems to be divine from the same reason that all the others do.

---

[1] A rather vast literature. In my brief synopsis here, I draw upon the more extensive study of *On the Sacred Disease* in Lloyd (1979) 15–29; 37–49. Subsequent authors,
such as Oberhelman (1990) and Prioreschi (1992), have been more insistent than Lloyd
about the ambiguity of distinctions between divine and natural developed by Hippocratic authors and others in the Greek rationalist medical tradition. Both Lloyd and
Oberhelman point to the seminal work of Edelstein in this area, although they modify
his views in various ways.

[2] A similar statement appears in *Airs, Waters, Places* (22.3–4 Diller). Although the
author of that treatise does not engage in an extended a criticism of belief in divine
causality as the author of *On the Sacred Disease*, he does deny the suggestion that
the disease 'Anarieis,' found among the Scythians, has any divine origin (22.4–7).
Furthermore, he makes the point that if the gods were involved in causing diseases, one
would expect the poor to suffer more than the rich, inasmuch as the poor cannot afford
as many or as costly sacrifices as the rich, and should therefore be more vulnerable to
divine anger; since this is not the case, however, the belief in divine causation of disease
is clearly false (22.8–10).

At the same time, he maintains that those who impute the cause of disease to the gods are in fact impious in asserting that the pure gods could or would cause disease (1.28; 1.44).[3] At the end of the treatise, the author expands upon his statement that all diseases are divine by remarking upon the divine nature of the universe as a whole:

> αὕτη δὲ ἡ νοῦσος ἡ ἱρὴ καλεομένη ἀπὸ τῶν αὐτῶν προφασίων γίνεται καὶ
> αἱ λοιπαί, ἀπὸ τῶν προσιόντων καὶ ἀπιόντων καὶ ψύχεος καὶ ἡλίου καὶ
> πνευμάτων μεταβαλλομένων τε καὶ οὐδέποτε ἀτρεμιζόντων. ταῦτα δ᾽ ἐστὶ
> θεῖα ὥστε μὴ δεῖν ἀποκρίνοντα τὸ νόσημα θειότερον τῶν λοιπῶν νομίζειν,
> ἀλλὰ πάντα θεῖα καὶ πάντα ἀνθρώπινα, φύσιν δὲ ἕκαστον ἔχει καὶ δύναμιν
> ἐφ᾽ ἑωυτοῦ, καὶ οὐδὲν ἄπορόν ἐστιν οὐδ᾽ ἀμήχανον.

> (18.1–2 Grensemann)

> This disease called sacred occurs from the same causes as other diseases —from things going in and exiting [the body] and from cold and the sun and from winds changing and never remaining undisturbed. These things are divine so that it is not necessary, setting the disease apart, to consider it more divine than the rest, but all are divine and all are human, and each has a nature and a power deriving from itself and none is incurable or untreatable.

In this passage, the author suggests that disease occurs as part of a divine necessity that governs all things. But his conception of 'divine nature' allows for the regularity and predictability of natural processes. As G.E.R. Lloyd writes, the author relies on 'the doctrine of the uniformity of nature, the regularity of causes and effects. If a factor is held to be a cause or contributory agent in bringing about disease, then the action of that factor must be supposed to be uniform.'[4] Indeed, the author is insistent that such processes are intelligible to the human mind; he asserts that if one can discover the cause of a disease, one can find an appropriate cure. His explanation of epilepsy depends upon the interaction between a particular kind of internal *physis* (an excessively phlegmatic constitution) and external environmental factors such as wind, water, heat and dryness; his cure involves keeping the affected

---

[3] The inverse remark, that humans cannot pollute the gods, is made by Theseus (*Her.* 1232) and Creon (*Ant.* 1042–1043).

[4] Lloyd (1979) 26; cf. Hankinson (1998) who, in an interpretation of this passage (together with *Aer.* 22), suggests that the Hippocratic model of disease causation does not so much reject the divine as relocate it: divinity is established as 'the very property of the world that renders it intelligible' (17). For other Hippocratic statements on the divine as a causative factor, cf. *Prog.* 1.19–22 and *Nat. Mul.* 1. Hankinson (1998: 23) argues that in these passages, too, the divine can be subsumed under the category of the natural, the grand scheme of the cosmos.

individual 'dry.' He is not so optimistic as to believe that medicine has already solved the specific puzzle of every disease, but he is confident that solutions will be found, using the sophisticated methods and logical thought-processes which he espouses. Certainly the unreliable techniques of charlatans and purifiers must be set aside in favor of the methods he advocates.

In addition to these attitudes regarding causality, it is important to remind ourselves of a significant difference between modern scientific and ancient Hippocratic conceptions of disease. Modern scientific medicine explains the spread of many diseases by reference to the concept of contagion (through proximity or physical contact), whereas Hippocratic authors resist the notion of contagion as a cause of disease while arguing in favor of meteorological and dietetic factors. Hippocratic authors divide diseases into two categories, epidemic and individual. The author of *Breaths* explains that *loimos* (plague) is due to bad air, and thus can infect whole populations; individuals can fall sick in the absence of plague because they practice a bad regimen. The air which causes plague contains some 'miasma,' the origins of which are unclear—certainly, the author of *Breaths* gives no explanation. The author does explain that a given plague does not inevitably infect everyone because individuals differ from one another in bodily constitution:

> ἔστιν δὲ δισσὰ ἔθνεα πυρετῶν, ὡς ταύτῃ διελθεῖν, ὁ μὲν κοινὸς ἅπασιν, ὁ καλεόμενος λοιμός, ὁ δὲ [διὰ πονηρὴν δίαιταν] ἰδίῃ τοῖσι πονηρῶς διαιτω-μένοισι γινόμενος. ἀμφοτέρων δὲ τούτων ὁ ἀὴρ αἴτιος. ὁ μὲν πολύκοινος πυρετὸς διὰ τοῦτο τοιοῦτός ἐστιν, ὅτι τὸ πνεῦμα τωὐτὸ πάντες ἕλκουσιν· ὁμοίου δὲ ὁμοίως τοῦ πνεύματος τῷ σώματι μιχθέντος, ὅμοιοι καὶ οἱ πυρε-τοὶ γίνονται. ἀλλ᾽ ἴσως φήσει τις· διὰ τί οὖν οὐχ ἅπασι τοῖσι ζῴοισιν, ἀλλ᾽ ἔθνει τινὶ αὐτῶν ἐπιπίπτουσιν αἱ τοιαῦται νοῦσοι; διότι διαφέρει, φαίην ἄν, καὶ σῶμα σώματος καὶ φύσις φύσιος καὶ τροφὴ τροφῆς. οὐ γὰρ πᾶσι τοῖσιν ἔθνεσιν τῶν ζῴων ταὐτὰ οὔτ᾽ ἀνάρμοστα οὔτ᾽ εὐάρμοστά ἐστιν, ἀλλ᾽ ἕτερα ἑτέροισι σύμφορα καὶ ἕτερα ἑτέροισιν ἀσύμφορα. ὅταν μὲν οὖν ὁ ἀὴρ τοι-ούτοισι χρωσθῇ μιάσμασιν, ἃ τῇ ἀνθρωπίνῃ φύσει πολέμιά ἐστιν, ἄνθρωποι τότε νοσέουσιν, ὅταν δὲ ἑτέρῳ τινὶ ἔθνει τῶν ζῴων ἀνάρμοστος ὁ ἀὴρ γένη-ται, κεῖνα τότε νοσέουσιν.   (6.1–2 Jouanna)

To proceed according to this view, there are two types of fevers, the one common to everyone, called plague, and the other arising individually in those people practicing poor regimen. But of both these types, air is the cause. The fever common to all is this way for the following reason: everyone takes in the same wind; and when a similar wind is mixed up in the body in a similar way, similar too will be the fevers arising. But perhaps someone will say: 'So then why do these diseases attack not all living creatures but only certain species of them?' Because, I would say,

body differs from body and nature from nature and sustenance from
sustenance. For the same things are neither poorly suited nor well suited
to every species of animals, but some things are appropriate for some
species and some are not appropriate. And so whenever the air is defiled
by such pollutions that are inimical to the nature of humans, it is humans
then who fall sick, but whenever the air becomes poorly suited to another
species of animals, then these creatures become sick.

The author of *Nature of Man* offers these same two categories of disease:
epidemics are again caused by bad air and individual diseases are due
to bad regimen (ch. 9). In this treatise, the air contains not a miasma,
but a νοσερὴ ἀπόκρισις ('a sickly secretion,' 9.5) which causes the disease. Again, the origins of this *apokrisis* are not explained. The author
also maintains that epidemic diseases can be avoided by escaping the
bad air through a *metastasis*, a change of location. The Hippocratic *Epidemics* do not specifically mention this form of disease causation, but
neither do they support the idea of contagion. Rather, the *katastaseis*,
particularly extensive in *Epidemics* 1 and 3, emphasize the various meteorological factors which the rationalist healers felt were sufficient explanation for the presence of widespread disease.

The Hippocratics are apparently alone in the fifth century in advocating this form of epidemic disease causation. So, for example, Thucydides maintains that the plague in Athens infected people all the more
when they came in close contact with one another (2.47.4, of the *iatroi*;
2.51.4, ἕτερος ἀφ' ἑτέρου θεραπείας ἀναπιμπλάμενοι ὥσπερ τὰ πρόβατα
ἔθνῃσκον, 'one person having been filled with the disease from another
through taking care of one another, so that they died like sheep'). Moreover, his discussion of the dogs and birds (2.50.1–2), while reminiscent
of details in the traditional plague stories handed down by poets, also
makes a significant point about contagion: only by eating the flesh of
the dead were the animals infected.[5] Indeed, he makes very little of the

---

[5] Demont (1983) argues that Thucydides mentions the facts about dogs and birds
in order to prove the abnormal and distinctive qualities of this plague to rationalist
members of his reading audience; Thucydides includes these details not only because
they were standard elements in plague descriptions, but also because he can counter
certain rationalist arguments with them: 'L'insistance rationelle de Thucydide se com-
prend aussi dans cette optique: il ne s'agit pas de convaincre la masse, qui, en restant à
la conception traditionelle attestée chez Hésiode, Homère, Hérodote, Sophocle, n'a nul
besoin d'une démonstration rationelle pour être convaincue de la portée universelle du
fléau; c'est la public informé et savant, qui risque de confondre des maladies dissem-
blables (la pestilence athénienne et les autres, à Lemnos et ailleurs, II, 47, 3), qu'il faut
convaincre par la raison du fait que ce λοιμός, cette pestilence, échappe aux catégories

meteorological situation[6]—and his description of the plague was later criticized by Galen as the work of an amateur (*De difficultate respirationis* 2.1, 7.850 Kühn). But Thucydides gives no support to traditional religious explanations for the cause of plague—the arrows of Apollo play no role in his description. At the same time, it is also true that contagion is an important element in the notion of pollution, certainly very much a part of traditional religious and social injunctions. Although the term for pollution, *miasma*, is in fact the very one used by the author of *Breaths* to describe the infecting elements contained in the air, pollution can be passed through human contact; moreover, the polluted individual is a clear source of infection, and must be shunned, expelled, purified, etc.[7] Scholars such as Mirko Grmek and Vivian Nutton stress that the Hippocratics seem to have been exceptional in rejecting the notion of contagion through contact; Nutton suggests that they may have moved away from the concept of contagion precisely because of its strong association with religious pollution.[8] By contrast, other sophisticated thinkers in antiquity may have set aside the role traditionally assigned to the gods in disease causation, but they retained the idea of contagion which was so important in religious explanations of pollution and disease.[9]

---

de l'art medical, puisque le mal ne limite pas ses effets aux hommes mais atteint par le contact alimentaire (notons que l'historien ne parle pas du rôle de l'air) les animaux qui dévorent les cadavres' (347).

[6] Although Demont points to some subtle hints in the text that suggest Thucydides was aware of standard medical explanations for plague, and that he does in fact include these: plague is associated by the medical writers with hot, dry air, and Demont argues that Thucydides not only mentions the geographical origins of the plague (in hot, dry Ethiopia, 2.48.1), but also much earlier describes three conditions (earthquakes, eclipses, and drought) under which the plague arose (1.23). See Demont (1983) 348–350.

[7] On pollution and contact, see extensive discussions in Parker (1983), e.g., 39–40, 49–54, 110.

[8] Grmek (1980a), Nutton (1983), esp. 1–16, and (2000). Scholars point to sources from the fifth and fourth centuries where the notion of contagion is clearly in operation: Isoc. *Aeg.* 390B 29; Plato *Phdr.* 255d; Soph. *OT* 179–181; decree from Kos, Sylloge no. 943 (cited by Demont [1983] 345 n. 13).

[9] These two conceptions of epidemic disease causation have interesting social consequences, according to Barbara Leavy. In her book, *To Blight with Plague: Studies in a Literary Theme* (New York 1992), the Hippocratic theory is designated as 'miasmatic' in contrast to the standard 'contagious' formulation. She argues, 'Both theories are morally charged. Miasma has to do with a world of widespread material corruption and as such it is easily translatable into a metaphor for the antithesis of civic virtue, which assumes the possibility for society to be organized for the well-being of its citizens' (24). Yet she points out that miasmatic theory (in the non-religious sense) removes responsibility from the individual and can act to unite a community against the myste-

If the medical healers do not envision deities visiting diseases on humans in some grand scheme of punishment, they nevertheless have their own set of factors which lie beyond human control and which influence the composition of the human body and its processes. The treatise *Airs, Waters, Places* describes how different winds, waters and geographical features effect different diseases and indeed different national characters. The Scythians are physically thick, moist, fleshy and homogeneous in appearance, because they live in a continually wet and chilly environment; the Asians are gentle yet tall and sturdy, with little variation in physique, because they live in a flourishing and evenly temperate climate; the Greeks, in keeping with the variety of their seasons and the differences in Greek terrain, are fierce, courageous, independent and diverse in size and shape. Yet the author is unwilling to assert that the environment is the sole force determining ethnic character and behavior. He argues that customs, particularly forms of government, can alter or sustain the characteristics imposed by the uncontrollable forces of nature (ch. 16). But it is clear that for the majority of Hippocratic physicians, the origins of disease can be found in the interplay between the individual's constitution, activities, and his or her natural environment.

Although the medical writers tend to agree that meteorology and geography are extremely influential factors in the health of a given population, they hardly speak with a consistent voice when it comes to analysis of the particulars. While the author of *Airs, Waters, Places* may argue that Asia is healthiest because of its temperate climate, he does not match up the specifics of wind, water and situation given in chapters 1–11 with the more general descriptions of national character and climate in 12–24. And even within his analysis of the effects of various waters, he is not consistent.[10] Furthermore, although Asia may be the healthiest place to live, it is not the best: Greece has that advantage because of the character of its people. The author of *Regimen*

---

rious intruder. By contrast, contagion theory is alienating and divisive, as fear of contracting the disease through contact leads to isolation: as Leavy writes 'communicable diseases intensify the isolation of individuals that eventually affects all social organization and relations' (18). Finally, she maintains that plagues in general induce a confrontation between the natural law of self-preservation and the divine and civic laws through which society organizes itself. Such a confrontation brings about the realization that 'however high a priority self-preservation may claim, it is also true that the body is a necessary but not sufficient criterion for self-hood' (39).

[10] See Diller (1934) 23–26.

2 also discusses climate, but, despite some correspondences, it is clear that this author does not rely on the author of *Airs, Waters, Places* for the particulars of climatology.[11] It seems almost impossible to find a healthy place to live from the facts presented by the author of *Regimen* in his climatological chapters (2.37–38). For example, the north wind appears on the whole to be healthier than the south (2.37.4), because the north wind is not naturally warm and dry; by contrast, the warm, dry south wind extracts moisture from the earth, the sea and all living things in an attempt to counteract its natural dryness (2.38.3–4). However, the north wind is naturally cold and wet—if excessively so, it can cause illness. Thus, the author maintains that mountain towns facing north are not healthy (2.37.4); yet neither are those that face south (2.37.3). Places deprived of the north wind are not healthy either, but islands out in the sea are better places in winter because they are not so affected by the cold coming in from the north. Any winds coming over the mountains provoke diseases, not only because they are dry, but also because they stir up the air which humans breathe (2.38.6). Thus, despite the many discussions of climatology in the Hippocratic Corpus, I am hard-pressed to find a climate that all the medical writers find truly healthy.

How much can we assume that the public (including the tragedians) knew about the theories debated among the medical thinkers? Xenophon's *Cyropaedia* provides some evidence for basic beliefs about health and health care at the height of the classical period. In the first book, Cyrus and his father have a wide-ranging discussion about the knowledge and practices necessary to a good ruler. At one point in the discussion (1.6.16), they begin to speak of military training. Cyrus refers to an earlier conversation in which his father maintained that a good general was not skilled in tactics alone, but also knew how to care for the health and well being of his army. Cyrus states that, in accordance with the recommendations of prominent military men, he has appointed healers to attend to the health of his army. In response, his father says that healers are fine for attending to those who are already sick, but that the general's job is to maintain the army's health—to practice, as it were, preventive medicine. To do so, one must attend to the location in which a camp is set up and to the health practices of the individual soldiers (1.6.16).[12] Next, Cyrus describes what he believes

---

[11] See the analysis of Joly in his commentary on *Regimen* 2.37–38.

[12] ἢν μὲν δήπου χρόνον τινὰ μέλλῃς ἐν τῷ αὐτῷ μένειν, ὑγιεινοῦ πρῶτον δεῖ στρατα-

to be a healthy regimen: one in which intake is balanced by expenditure (1.6.17).[13] The essential concerns in this passage are geographic factors and dietary concerns—the impact of the environment and the lifestyle of the individual. As we shall see, tragedy, too, reflects the basic notions of disease causation and control found here in the *Cyropaedia*, as it explores the relationship between individual responsibility and environmental influences, broadly understood.

τοπέδου μὴ ἀμελῆσαι· τούτου δὲ οὐκ ἂν ἁμάρτοις, ἐάνπερ μελήσῃ σοι. καὶ γὰρ λέγοντες οὐδὲν παύονται ἄνθρωποι περί τε τῶν νοσηρῶν χωρίων καὶ περὶ τῶν ὑγιεινῶν· μάρτυρες δὲ σαφεῖς ἑκατέροις αὐτῶν παρίστανται τά τε σώματα καὶ τὰ χρώματα. ἔπειτα δὲ οὐ τὰ χωρία μόνον ἀρκέσει σκέψασθαι, ἀλλὰ μνήσθητι σὺ πῶς πειρᾷ σαυτοῦ ἐπιμέλεσθαι ὅπως ὑγιαίνῃς. ('If in fact you intend to remain in the same place for a certain period of time, it is necessary first of all not to neglect the health of the encampment; and you would not make a mistake if this is a concern for you. For people do not stop talking about unhealthy locations and healthy ones: and there are clear witnesses for each of these things at hand as far as both bodies and complexions go. So then it will be fitting to consider not only the location, but also you should remember to try to take care of yourself, so that you will stay healthy.')

[13] καὶ ὁ Κῦρος εἶπε, πρῶτον μὲν νὴ Δία πειρῶμαι μηδέποτε ὑπερπίμπλασθαι· δύσφορον γάρ· ἔπειτα δὲ ἐκπονῶ τὰ εἰσιόντα· οὕτω γάρ μοι δοκεῖ ἥ τε ὑγίεια μᾶλλον παραμένειν καὶ ἰσχὺς προσγενέσθαι. ('And Cyrus said, "First by Zeus I try never to eat too much; for that is oppressive; then I work off what I take in; for in this way it seems to me that health will persist and increase in strength."')

CHAPTER FIVE

REMEDY IN THE HIPPOCRATIC CORPUS

If we now turn to consider methods of healing, the lack of clear consensus and consistency among the Hippocratics on the issue of remedy will become immediately apparent. Furthermore, there are often significant gaps between theory and practice. Indeed, many authors, when they turn to give therapeutic advice, seem much more concerned with the actions and reactions of the individual patient—the universal generalities are often qualified when the healer is confronted by a particular patient.[1] But data drawn from clinical practice is rarely allowed to disrupt the basic theoretical foundations. The healer will simply add the symptoms and reactions of a new patient to what he has already experienced with former patients.[2]

This does not mean that the authors never disagreed with one another. While healers were proud of their profession, they recognized differences among the ranks. Thus, although the author of *Regimen in Acute Diseases* is quite confident in his own ability to treat disease, he nevertheless acknowledges the contrary prescriptions advanced by different members of the profession (7), even when they are working from the same essential belief in the power of regimen to heal the sick. He argues that regimen is the best form of therapy: 'it has great power to bring all the sick to health, to secure the condition of the healthy, to bring the athlete to peak condition, and to grant whatever any person wants' (καὶ γὰρ τοῖσι νοσέουσι πᾶσιν ἐς ὑγιείην μέγα τι δύναται καὶ τοῖσιν ὑγιαίνουσιν ἐς ἀσφάλειαν καὶ τοῖσιν ἀσκέουσιν ἐς εὐεξίην καὶ ἐς ὅ τι ἕκαστος θέλει, 9). He goes on to extol the virtues of barley-gruel in no uncertain terms (10; 15). Yet several chapters later, we find the author indicating that in fact barley-gruel is not good in all cases (16). To be sure, the author treats his ability to modify the remedy according to

---

[1] The authors of the Hippocratic Corpus thus anticipate the Aristotelian argument that rules and theories of nature are valid if they hold 'for the most part' (ὡς ἐπὶ τὸ πολύ), such that individual exceptions can be accomodated. On this issue, cf. von Staden (2002).

[2] Cf. the remarks of Langholf (1990: 212) on the 'additive nature' of Greek medicine.

the circumstances of the particular patient as a virtue—and no doubt
it is. But the qualifications do tend to undercut the glowing report on
barley-gruel first advanced by the author. Furthermore, the author's
idealized praise of regimen is surely undercut by the very treatise that
he is writing, a treatise which admits of disagreement, failure, and the
on-going battle with disease; if regimen has the power to give each
person what he desires, it has certainly failed to do so thus far.

The numerous remedial recipes proffered in various treatises may
attest to the healer's ability to cure disease; they show that he has the
tools of treatment. In the gynecological treatises, the very multiplicity
of remedies which are directed at cleansing, moistening, and softening the uterus may suggest the healer's inability to provide a consistent
and reliable cure for infertility, but, of course, it may also suggest the
healer's actual ability to respond with flexibility to the cases presented
by different patients. These remedies, which include such substances as
hellebore, wine, squill, dung, myrrh, cantharid beetles, oil, beaver testi-
cles, and copper particles, are rather daunting for the modern reader.
Moreover, a number of the gynecological treatises present the remedies simply in lists: 'a remedy for …,' 'another remedy for …,' 'another
remedy for … .'[3] These lists often make no attempt to link the remedy
to a particular type of patient, or to specify when the remedy should
not be used. They may thereby suggest to us a random or haphazard therapeutics, based not on knowledge or theory, but on hope. But
the modern reader is no doubt less susceptible to the power of the
catalogue, which oral theorists have argued is an important source of
authority and control in non-literate societies.[4] Even though Greece of
the late fifth century can hardly be termed a non-literate society, the
power and the traditions of orality were still very strong.[5] At the same
time, the Hippocratics were clearly interested in what writing down
their findings might offer to the medical community: as Philip van der
Eijk has argued in a wide-ranging discussion of the rhetorical structures

---

[3] See examples of this style in (e.g.) *Superf.* 33.8–9, 11–13; 35; 37; 39.

[4] Cf. Vansina (1985); see also Taylor (2000) for a discussion of the function of lists
in early Greece, especially in the development of a Greek sense of history. Grmek
(1989: 92) writes that the effect of Hippocratic medicine on public health was 'merely
psychological'; but that psychology may have been significant to the Greeks' sense of
control over their health.

[5] For an initial inquiry into the issue of catalogues in the Hippocratic Corpus, see
Smith (1983). For the continuing importance of oral transmission of medical information, see Van der Eijk (1997) 95–97.

and practices of Hippocratic treatises, the Hippocratics came to understand that the production of written records would provide 'a common
reservoir of knowledge accessible to a group of physicians … and admitting of additions and changes by this same group of physicians.' Furthermore, he argues that they saw the written record not merely as
an instrument for storing knowledge but also for 'keep[ing] knowledge
available for practical application.'[6] Van der Eijk suggests that the catalogues of diseases and remedies are structured to allow for the easy
inclusion of new information as it arises.[7]

Research done in recent decades also indicates that these lists of
remedies are based on certain methodological and theoretical principles.[8] Georg Harig has analyzed the pharmacology of a number of treatises,[9] providing a helpful list of the qualities attributed by the authors to
different 'simples,' which were the plants or foods themselves, unmixed
with any other elements; the authors are primarily interested in the
cooling, warming, wetting, or drying capabilities of the recommended
substances. Unfortunately, the authors do not always agree on the properties of a substance,[10] nor do they always explain their reasoning. Only
Regimen draws more complex lessons from the nature of the various substances it recommends, attempting to align the taste and feel of a food
with its medicinal qualities.[11] For example, the author writes at 2.56

---

[6] Van der Eijk (1997) 98.

[7] Van der Eijk (1997) 112. Greek medical papyri (e.g., the Michigan Medical Codex)
attest to the enduring nature of various remedies, to which new information is added,
but 'nothing seems to have been subtracted' (Hanson's introduction in Youtie [1996]
xix).

[8] One might argue that the empirical nature of the actual practice of medicine in
this period would not permit remedies to endure had they had noticeably detrimental
effects. This is not a particularly strong argument: consider the persistence of certain
practices such as bleeding, which continued into the twentieth century (this is not to
say that bleeding is invariably harmful and is in fact important for the control of
some diseases such as hemachromatosis; for a discussion of some beneficial aspects
of bleeding, see Brain [1986] ch. 10). Furthermore, there is in Hippocratic medicine
the above-mentioned tendency not to delete remedies found unhelpful, but rather to
add on new corrective information (see notes 2 and 7). See the discussion in Hanson
(1991), where she analyzes the fate of three traditional types of remedy in the hands of
Hippocratic healers.

[9] Harig (1980). He discusses *Regimen, Affections, Diseases 3, Ulcers, Regimen in Acute
Diseases, Epidemics 6,* and *Places in Man.*

[10] See examples in Harig (1980) 230–232. He observes, e.g, that *Regimen* considers
lentils to be burning whereas *Epidemics* 6 describes them as cooling; *Regimen* characterizes basil as drying, whereas *Affections* describes it as wet and cold.

[11] Although the author of *On Ancient Medicine* believes that the healer must understand this complex character of different foods and drugs, arguing that such qualities

that what is sweet, sharp, salty, bitter, compact and fleshy is warming; material which has these qualities but is also dry warms and dries; similarly, that which consists of these basic qualities, but is wetter, warms and moistens.[12] The treatises *Ulcers*, *Fistulas*, and *Hemorrhoids* list many different drug combinations which may appear haphazard or at any rate horrifying to the modern reader. However, the research of John Scarborough has demonstrated that many of these remedies do have a basic theoretical underpinning, and it is an allopathic one. Scarborough shows, for example, that the remedies given in chapter 11 of *Ulcers* are all intended to dry out the wound/ulcer, which is considered wet.[13]

Any discussion of therapeutics must no doubt make mention of the two doctrinal orientations in Hippocratic medicine that seem to have developed during the fifth century: dietetics, which focused on preventive medicine, and the more traditional approaches of pharmacology and surgery, now recast in a sophisticated mold. Dietetics certainly finds antecedents in Homer, Hesiod and, above all, the precepts ascribed to Pythagoras.[14] And many discussions regarding particular characteristics of foods, herbs, and daily habits share the findings and assumptions of pharmacology and surgery. But dietetics differed from these other forms of medicine in asserting its ability to prevent disease from occurring at all. Like other traditions of sophisticated medicine, dietetics operated in the belief that health was achieved through the equilibrium of bodily elements, but healers in the dietetic business placed greater emphasis on health maintenance than on the expulsion of disease from the body. Dietetics is thus a more empowering brand of medical practice than that offered by those who practiced cautery, surgery, and pharmacology, in that it gives the individual the ability to control the health of his own body.[15] But, as scholars point out, dietetics also

---

as sharp, sweet, smooth, etc. are more important than the basic hot/cold/warm/dry categorizations, he does not engage in the kind of extensive description of individual foods which the author of *Regimen* 2 supplies.

   [12] Harig (1980: 236–239) gives some examples of partially and diametrically opposed evaluations of a number of different substances.

   [13] Scarborough (1983), with discussion of *Ulcers* 11 on pp. 318–323.

   [14] Wöhrle (1990) 18–49. He also discusses under the rubric of 'Zwei Archegeten' the history and reputation ascribed to Herodicus of Selymbria (c. 500–430/20 BCE) and Iccus of Tarentum (5th century). Herodicus was particularly renowned for prescriptions on dietetics which he made in his role as an athletic trainer; Iccus, also an athletic trainer, was known for prescribing restrictions on the sexual activity of his charges (Wöhrle, 49–59).

   [15] Edelstein (1931/1967), especially 304. Edelstein notes that philosophers such as

operates on basic notions common to all Hippocratic medicine: not only is the belief in equilibrium essential, but also the notion that disease arises from *plêthôra* (the amassing of too much of a humor in one place) or *kenôsis* (the lack of a humor and the resulting *horror vacui*).[16] Moreover, the reality of disease inevitably plays a role in dietetic treatises, for even the most careful patients were subject to illness; thus, the rationalist healers tried to develop regimens which would not only prevent disease but would also cure it.

The dietetic approach to healing introduces another fundamental issue in medicine, which concerns the ability of the body to heal itself. In his important study on the different notions of *pharmaka* operative in early Greek culture, Artelt places the use of *pharmaka* in the allopathic[17] tradition of medicine and dietetics in the tradition of 'biologische Heilkunst'—that is, the ability of the body to heal itself.[18] The idea of an *automatos* (self-regulating, spontaneous) healing process appears explicitly only in a few Hippocratic texts. The author of the *Appendix to Regimen in Acute Diseases* advises against drug therapy in some circumstances, because it is possible to disrupt the natural healing process; after a list of certain symptoms, he writes: τῶν τοιῶνδε μηδένα φαρμακεύειν. κίνδυνόν τε γὰρ ἕξει καὶ οὐδὲν ὠφελήσεις τάς τε ἀπὸ τοῦ αὐτομάτου κρισίας ἀφαιρήσεις (55 Potter: 'Do not use drug therapy for these. For it will be dangerous and you will provide no help and you will prevent the *krises* from happening spontaneously').[19] The author of *On Ancient Medicine* illustrates the body's ability to heal itself by pointing

---

Plato were particularly disturbed by the dietetic brand of medicine, because it led the individual to concentrate far too much on the health of his body, and far too little on the health of his soul (313–314).

[16] See discussions in Lorenz (1990) 273–274, and Lonie (1981) 113, 266–268. Lonie remarks on the prevalence of belief that εὐρυχωρίαι (wide open spaces) will inevitably attract substances to them on the *horror vacui* principle (especially elucidated later by Erasistratus) and Lorenz makes a more general statement on Hippocratic concepts of sickness and health when he writes, 'Härte, Undurchlässigkeit, Anschoppung, Verstopfung waren die vorherrschenden Modelle der Pathologenese, Lockerung, Durchbruch, und Lösung (Lysis) jene der Heilung' (326–327).

[17] Allopathy is the process of healing through opposites (e.g., heat cured by cold); see further below in section a.

[18] Artelt (1937) 54, with further discussion on the power of the body to heal itself and the appropriate use of *pharmaka* on 55–67.

[19] Of course, treatises exist which give completely the opposite advice, arguing that it is exactly when the body is ill and weakened by strong diseases that it need drugs the most: so *Loc. Hom.* 43, 45. See more below in section on '*malthakia* and *ischys.*'

out how chills are healed by fever. He ends this particular segment of his argument with an appeal to the commonality of allopathic healing processes in the body, asking rhetorically:

> ᾧ οὖν διὰ τάχεος οὕτω παραγίνεται τὸ ἐναντιώτατόν τε καὶ ἀφαιρεόμενον τὴν δύναμιν ἀπὸ ταὐτομάτου, τί ἂν ἀπὸ τούτου μέγα ἢ δεινὸν γένοιτο; ἢ τί δεῖ πολλῆς ἐπὶ τοῦτο βοηθείης;   (16.8 Jouanna)

> And so what great or terrible thing could arise from that thing to which the most opposite arises, spontaneously depriving it of power? What need is there of great help against this?

Nevertheless, the author of this treatise expends a great deal of effort arguing for the existence of and the need for the medical arts; thus, his words here are no recommendation against medical treatment or derogation of medicine itself. Rather, he is concerned to demonstrate that nature itself shows the way to healing, giving clues which intelligent men can pick up and develop into consistent forms of remedy. Healers are necessary when the disease is too strong for the body to handle through the resources of its own nature. *Internal Affections* provides an example which incorporates both the idea of automatic healing and the power of medicine: the author gives a set of symptoms and then writes, τούτῳ ἢν μὲν ἡ γαστὴρ αὐτομάτη ταραχθῇ, ἐγγυτάτω ὑγιὴς προβαίνει. ἢν οὖν μὴ ταραχθῇ αὐτομάτη ἡ κοιλίη, καθαίρειν χρὴ διδόντα ... (21: 'if the stomach of this patient is moved spontaneously [i.e., cleaned out], he is coming very near to being healthy. But if the belly is not moved spontaneously, it is necessary to clean it out, giving ...' [a list of remedies follows]).[20]

In addition to this distinction between dietetic and pharmacological approaches to health and healing, three other major areas of contention appear in medical approaches to remedy, which for the sake of convenience I will give the labels allopathy, *metabolê* (change), and *apostasis* (expulsion). A further issue requiring analysis to some extent fits all of these categories: it is the problem of degrees—that is, healers discuss

---

[20] The odd usage of ταραχθῇ in a positive sense should be noted; however, it seems that the disturbance of the stomach must take place on the road to healing; thus, it is a sign that the patient will get better. Elsewhere in *Internal Affections*, the use of the verb *tarattein* is clearly negative (cf., e.g., ch. 39).

On the notion of *automatos* healing, see also the use of the idea in *Diseases of Women* 2.116, where it occurs in conjunction with the notion of good luck:... ἢν μή τι εὐτύχημα τῶν αὐτομάτων λύσῃ γενόμενον ('unless some good luck arising spontaneously should provide relief'). Cf. also *Morb.* 1.7, *Decent.* 6.

the potential benefits and injuries of 'strong' and 'weak' therapies. Hippocratic discussions of remedy often combine these principles in various ways, but for the purposes of clarity, I will try to give separate overviews of each one.

a. *Allopathy*

A central tenet recurring in Hippocratic texts is that disease can be cured by using the principle of allopathy (*contraria contrariis curantur*, 'opposites are cured by opposites'). The predominance of the allopathic principle is perhaps not surprising when seen in the larger context of Greek speculative thought, in which the nature of the world was so often expressed in terms of polar oppositions: from the Pythagoreans to Heraclitus to Empedocles, from Protagoras and Anaxagoras to Plato and Aristotle, from Homer and Hesiod to the tragedians and the historians of the fifth century, oppositional structures characterize the world view presented therein. Such oppositional thinking can be discerned in many areas of Hippocratic therapeutics: some authors urge the use of strong medicines to counteract strong diseases; some authors argue that the violent changes suffered in acute diseases must be counteracted swiftly by attempts to change the course in the opposite direction—if the affected person has been following one regimen, they must change to a different one; other treatises maintain that the healer must counteract the misbehavior of humors in the body—the person suffering under the influence of too much phlegm must be dried out and warmed up, whereas the excessively bilious should be cooled off and watered down. Yet the general principle is not so easily applied to practical treatment: is a strong medicine the opposite of a strong disease or is it the same because both are strong (and the patient would thus suffer all the more from the effects of two violent forces at work)? Perhaps a gentle medicine is the opposite of a strong disease. Again, do swift change (*metabolê*) and drastic measures really counteract the changes in the body due to disease or do these merely render the body just as unstable from different causes? How does one decide whether a particular treatment or drug is 'warm' or 'cold' or 'dry' or 'wet'? Establishing true opposites can be very difficult. To take a non-medical example, what is the answer to the question, 'Who is the opposite of the King?' Is the answer 'the Queen,' or is it, 'a commoner'? Neither answer is wrong, but is one more valid than the other?

G.E.R. Lloyd has argued that there was a strong tendency in the fifth century to treat all opposites as either 'incompatible' or 'exhaustive,' stating that it is only in the later dialogues of Plato that we begin to see changes in the 'unquestioned assumption that such pairs of opposites as one and many, being and not-being, are necessarily incompatible and exhaustive alternatives.'[21] Lloyd believes that 'Plato himself was responsible for drawing important distinctions between different types of opposites, for clarifying the problem of contradiction and in particular, for showing that apparently contradictory statements in which a thing is asserted both to be (in some sense) and not to be (in some other sense) are not contradictions at all.'[22] Plato and Aristotle may have been able to provide solutions to the problems vexing their predecessors, yet we should not suppose that earlier thinkers had not recognized the problem of different modes of opposition at all. The author of *On Ancient Medicine* makes a particularly strong case against what he sees are the problems of logic and of practicality in the theories of his fellow physicians. He criticizes those who apply the principle of opposites based on a very limited range of elemental substances; he maintains that there is a wide range of substances which combine in different ways within the body (13–15). Moreover, he is dissatisfied with the emphasis on theory that he finds in the works of his contemporaries (especially at the beginning of 15: ἀπορέω δ᾽ ἔγωγε οἱ τὸν λόγον ἐκεῖνον λέγοντες καὶ ἄγοντες ἐκ ταύτης τῆς ὁδοῦ ἐπὶ ὑπόθεσιν τὴν τέχνην τίνα ποτὲ τρόπον θεραπεύουσι τοὺς ἀνθρώπους ὥσπερ ὑποτίθενται … ['I myself am at a loss, with regard to those making this argument and bringing the *technê* through this line of reasoning to a hypothesis, as to how they treat people according to what they hypothesize']). The author of *Breaths* argues that air, utterly essential for living, is at same time the cause of diseases in the body; air, he maintains, can introduce pollutants into the body (5.1) or can itself act disruptively once inside the body (7.1ff.); air is thus the cause of the healthy being healthy and the sick being sick (4.1). The difficulty lies in going from theory to practice. If air is the cause of both sickness and health, how and where does one find a counteragent for air? After all, one cannot simply stop breathing.[23] Similarly, the author of *Regimen* may well argue that dis-

---

[21] Lloyd (1966) 127.

[22] Lloyd (1966) 127.

[23] Although the author of *Nature of Man* recommends something close to this when discussing the treatment of epidemic diseases (spread by air, he believes). At the end

ease results from a disequilibrium of the fundamental substances, fire and water, from which the body is composed; he further suggests that disease can be cured by counteracting excessive fire or excessive water with their respective opposites (*Reg.* 1. 32 and 33).[24] But, the author of *On Ancient Medicine* might object, there are again problems when it comes to the application of the theory: we cannot eat fire, after all, nor is water, even of the purest kind, a reliable cure for fever. Even if one argues for a base of four properties, consisting of hot, cold, wet, and dry, there are objections: if a man, diagnosed as suffering from 'cold,' is told to take something 'warm,' he will no doubt ask, 'what?' (15). The author of *Regimen* does provide an answer to this in the second two books of his treatise, where he lists all sort of foods and food mixtures as either cooling, wetting, heating, or drying (and various combinations thereof).

Despite their own awareness of such problems arising in discussions of both causation and therapeutics, the Hippocratic authors were not able to translate their techniques into effective and new formulations of the theory of opposites. Rather, allopathic theory remained to some extent divorced from the day-to-day therapeutics undertaken by the healer.

Let us look a little more closely at texts wherein theoretical principles of therapeutics are discussed. The allopathic principle is stated most clearly by the author of *Breaths*: τὰ ἐναντία τῶν ἐναντίων ἐστὶν ἰήματα (1.5: 'opposites are the cures for opposites'). These words are seconded either explicitly or implicitly in a number of other texts.[25] However,

---

of ch. 9, he writes τοῦ δὲ πνεύματος ὅπως ἡ ῥύσις ὡς ἐλαχίστη ἐς τὸ σῶμα ἐσίῃ καὶ ὡς ξεινοτάτη προμηθεῖσθαι, τῶν τε χωρίων τοὺς τόπους μεταβάλλοντα ἐς δύναμιν, ἐν οἷσιν ἂν ἡ νοῦσος καθεστήκῃ, καὶ τὰ σώματα λεπτύνοντα· οὕτω γὰρ ἂν ἥκιστα πολλοῦ τε καὶ πυκνοῦ τοῦ πνεύματος χρῄζοιεν οἱ ἄνθρωποι. ('Care should be taken that the amount of air breathed should be as small as possible and as unfamiliar as possible. These points may be dealt with by making the body thin so that the patient will avoid large and frequent breaths, and whenever practicable, by a change of station from the infected area' [trans. Chadwick and Mann]).

[24] Chapter 32 concerns the constitution of the body, 33, the constitution of the soul.

[25] E.g., *On Ancient Medicine*, beginning a critique of the 'theory group' of physicians: ἐπὶ δὲ τὸν τῶν τὸν καινὸν τρόπον τὴν τέχνην ζητεύντων ἐξ ὑποθέσιος λόγον ἐπανελθεῖν βούλομαι. εἰ γάρ τί ἐστιν θερμὸν ἢ ψυχρὸν ἢ ξηρὸν ἢ ὑγρὸν τὸ λυμαινόμενον τὸν ἄνθρωπον, καὶ δεῖ τὸν ὀρθῶς ἰητρεύοντα βοηθεῖν τῷ μὲν θερμῷ ἐπὶ τὸ ψυχρόν, τῷ δὲ ψυχρῷ ἐπὶ τὸ θερμόν, τῷ δὲ ξηρῷ ἐπὶ τὸ ὑγρόν, τῷ δὲ ὑγρῷ ἐπὶ τὸ ξηρόν, ... (13: 'The reasoning of those seeking through hypothesis the new method with respect to *technê* I wish to go through. For if there is something hot or cold or dry or wet harming humankind, and

certain texts seem to bring up the possibility of homeopathic remedy. C.W. Müller has shown that two oft-cited examples of homeopathic remedial theory in the Hippocratic Corpus—*On the Sacred Disease* 18 and *Places in Man* 42—have been poorly understood by scholars, who have ignored the context in which these statements are made. In *On the Sacred Disease*, it is stated that ἀκεστά τε τὰ πλεῖστά ἐστι τοῖς αὐτοῖσι τούτοισιν ἀφ᾿ ὧν καὶ γίνεται (18.3: 'most things are susceptible to healing by the same things from which they have arisen'). Müller demonstrates that the author of *On the Sacred Disease*, who clearly works on the basis of an allopathic system of remedy in the rest of his treatise, does not mean that diseases should be cured by the very same things which caused them, but rather that diseases arise from natural causes, and can therefore be cured by remedies found in nature. This author, who is so optimistic as to think that all diseases are curable once their natural causes are understood (18.2), is therefore opposing natural to supernatural; he is not advocating a homeopathic system of remedy. Similarly, the author of *Places in Man* seems to support homeopathic principles in 42:

> πυρετὸς ὁ διὰ φλεγμασίην γινόμενος, τοτὲ μὲν ὑπὸ τῶν αὐτῶν γίνεται καὶ παύεται, τοτὲ δὲ τοῖσιν ὑπεναντίοισι ⟨παύεται⟩ ἢ ⟨οἷσιν⟩ ἐγένετο. ... καὶ εἰ μὲν οὕτως εἶχε πᾶσι, καθεστήκει ἄν, οὕτω τὰ μὲν τοῖσον ὑπεναντίοισιν εὐτρεπίζεσθαι οἷά τέ ἐστι καὶ ἀφ᾿ ὅτου ἐγένετο, τὰ δὲ τοῖσιν ὁμοίοισιν οἷά τέ ἐστι καὶ ἀφ᾿ ὅτου ἐγένετο.   (42.3, 42.4 Craik)

> Fever arising on account of a phlegmatic condition sometimes begins and ends by the same things, but sometimes is stopped by opposites to those from which it arose. ... And if it held true in all cases, it would be established that some things are able to be cured by things that are opposite to those from which they arose, and other things can be treated by the things that are similar to those from which they arose.

However, Müller points out that the author of *Places in Man* mentions the potential effectiveness of homeopathic cures because he is concerned to show that no single overarching principle of therapeutics can suffice; rather, the art of medicine requires that the physician learn through experience when to treat by means of *ta homoia* (similars), when by *ta enantia* (opposites) and when by a combination of both. Müller argues convincingly that the author of *Places in Man* is far less interested

---

it is necessary that the person treating correctly help using heat against cold or cold against heat, or wet against dry, ...'); cf. *Aph.* 2.22; *Nat. Hom.* 9.1–2 and 13.

in the actual merits of homeopathic therapeutics than he is in asserting the importance of empiricism for medical *technê*.[26]

But while Müller sets out good arguments for downplaying or even dismissing the force or significance of homeopathic theory in these texts, there are still other treatises in which the principle of homeopathy is in evidence. The *Nature of Man*, which advances the allopathic principle of remedy in Chapters 9 and 13, nevertheless puts forth a homeopathic explanation of how drugs actually function in the body:

> τὸ γὰρ φάρμακον, ὅταν ἐσέλθῃ ἐς τὸ σῶμα, πρῶτον μὲν ἄγει ὃ ἂν αὐτῷ κατὰ φύσιν μάλιστα ᾖ τῶν ἐν τῷ σώματι ἐνεόντων, ἔπειτα δὲ καὶ τἆλλα ἕλκει τε καὶ καθαίρει. ὡς γὰρ τὰ φυόμενά τε καὶ σπειρόμενα, ὁπόταν ἐς τὴν γῆν ἔλθῃ, ἕλκει ἕκαστον τὸ κατὰ φύσιν αὐτῷ ἐνεὸν ἐν τῇ γῇ ...
>
> (6.3 Jouanna)

> For the drug, whenever it enters into the body, first brings out whatever is particularly similar to it of those things in the body, and then it draws out and cleanses the rest. For just as plants and seeds, whenever they go into the earth, each draws the thing in the earth which is naturally suited to it ...

Moreover, the homeopathic principle is clearly at work in a small number of remedies found in gynecological treatises, where recipes call for the use of feces and dirt in addition to the more usual range of substances (wine, herbs, honey, etc.).[27] Because this concept of Drekapotheke is not used in remedies given to males, it seems reasonable to connect the use of dirty substances with the 'dirt' of women's menstrual blood. Although it may be argued that such remedies derive from traditional medicine and were not actually developed by Hippocratic healers, the willingness of these very healers to repeat those remedies shows that the homeopathic way of thinking runs deep—especially when dealing with such potentially dangerous and unclean substances as women's menstrual blood.[28]

---

[26] Müller (1965b).

[27] See analysis in von Staden (1992a).

[28] Arguing against a *similia similibus* interpretation for the use of these substances in Hippocratic medicine, Ann Hanson prefers to see the persistence of dirty substances in the gynecological treatises as deriving from the Hippocratic interest in promoting fertility. She suggests that 'the excrement and urine seemed to be "fertilizers" (on analogy with Earth) or "cosmetics" (cf. the continued use of excrement as a "softening agent" and a stimulant for the growth of hair, in particular—and thus feeding back into the notions that these are fertilizers).' (personal communication, May 4, 1994); see further in Hanson (1998) 89, where she argues that the 'contextualization [of these

Homeopathy is in fact no stranger to Greek thought patterns, despite the prevalence of the *contraria contrariis* principle in Greek philosophy. The story of Telephus, who can only be healed by Achilles, the man who harmed him, exemplifies the power of homeopathic thinking in myth. Moreover, the *similia similibus* principle is often operative in Greek magic (and indeed, magic in other cultures as well).[29] The ability of like to attract and influence like was a fundamental Greek belief, found even in the earliest literary sources.[30] Indeed, Hippocratic authors utilize this principle to explain a whole range of issues, ranging from disease causation to the growth of the human body. For example, the author of *Nature of the Child* begins his explanation of embryonic growth with the words: ἔρχεται ἐν αὐτῇ ἕκαστον τὸ ὅμοιον ὡς τὸ ὅμοιον ... καὶ ἕκαστον ἔρχεται ἐς χώρην ἰδίην κατὰ τὸ συγγενές, ἀφ᾽ οὗ καὶ ἐγένετο, ... (17.1: 'each similar part in it goes to its similar part, ... and each goes to its own place according to the related part, from which it arose ...').[31] The attraction of like humors to one another is also essential to theories propounded in other texts. Thus, the ability of food both to harm and to help results, it is said, from homeopathy: food contains within it the different bodily forces[32] or humors,[33] and, in the process

---

substances] in the midst of medicaments that conformed to the mechanical paradigms of curing through opposites tempered the force of their messages.'

[29] Cf. Faraone (1991) who notes the importance of the *similia similibus* principle in magic; see esp. pp. 5–10.

[30] So Homer, *Odyssey* 17. 218 ὡς αἰεὶ τὸν ὁμοῖον ἄγει θέος ὡς τὸν ὁμοῖον ('so god always leads like to like').

[31] See discussion in Lonie (1981) 176–187 and cf. Müller (1965a). Lonie gives two examples found in Presocratic philosophy: Anaxagoras (DK59 A41): ἐκεῖνος γάρ φησιν ἐν τῇ διακρίσει τοῦ ἀπείρου τὰ συγγενῆ φέρεσθαι πρὸς ἄλληλα ('for he says that in the differentiation of the land related things were borne towards each other') and Democritus (DK68 A38): πεφυκέναι γὰρ τὸ ὅμοιον ὑπὸ τοῦ ὁμοίου κινεῖσθαι καὶ φέρεσθαι τά συγγενῆ πρὸς ἄλληλα ('for similar things are naturally moved by similar ones and related things are naturally borne towards one another').

[32] That is, the *dynamia* of *On Ancient Medicine* (esp. ch. 14) and *Regimen* 1–3.

[33] The author of *Nature of the Child* goes on to elaborate a homeopathic theory of nutrition and disease causation in *Diseases* 4, when he states that ἐν τοῖσι βρωτοῖσι καὶ τοῖσι ποτοῖσιν ἔνεστι πᾶσι καὶ χολώδεός τι καὶ ὑδρωποειδέος καὶ αἱματώδεος καὶ φλεγματώδεος, τῇ μὲν πλέον, τῇ δὲ ἔλασσον ... Ἔπην δὲ φάγῃ ἢ πίῃ ὁ ἄνθρωπος, ἕλκει τὸ σῶμα ἐς ἑωυτὸ ἐκ τῆς κοιλίης τῆς ἰκμάδος τῆς εἰρημένης ... ἡ ὁμοίη ἰκμὰς τὴν ὁμοίην, καὶ διαδίδωσι τῷ σώματι, ὥσπερ ἐπὶ τῶν φυτῶν ἕλκει ἀπὸ τῆς γῆς ἡ ὁμοίη ἰκμὰς τὴν ὁμοίην (33.2–3: 'all foods and drinks contain a greater or a lesser quantity of bilious, watery, bloody, or phlegmatic substance ... Now, whenever a man eats or drinks anything, the body attracts to itself the humour I have mentioned from the stomach, ... Each kind of humor attracts its like, and distributes it to the body, just as in the case of plants each kind of humour attracts its like' [trans. Lonie]).

of digestion, each humor moves to join the like humor already situated in the body. However, foods differ with respect to the proportions of the various humors they contain; thus, every act of eating is potentially dangerous, as the food may introduce too much of a particular humor, which will in turn disrupt the body's equilibrium. Homeopathic processes can therefore be both productive and destructive; they are necessary to human growth, strength, and health maintenance, yet they can also result in excess within the body, a major cause of disease.[34]

b. Metabolê

Often closely linked with the principle of allopathy, the concept of *metabolê* (change) arises in various contexts throughout the Corpus. It is a term used to describe internal changes in the body resulting from the onset of disease and changes in the course or type of disease; it can also describe changing external factors, such as variations in regimen, medical treatment or the weather.[35] If change has resulted in sickness, it is the healer's task to counteract or reverse the direction of the change in order to restore health. Thus the term *metabolê* turns up in discussions of causation, pathology, and treatment.[36] Many Hippocratic authors maintain that a patient's health can be improved by a change in diet/regimen, a change which either runs counter to the patient's normal habits or at least opposes the specific cause of the disease (contained in something the patient ate or breathed). Change is bad for the healthy man or woman, but necessary for the sick. But the healers do

---

[34] Guardasole (2000) gives a succinct account of the homeopathy/allopathy issue in tragedy; she cites Sophocles fr. 854 Radt (*incert. fab.*) πικρὰν πικρῷ κλύζουσι (*sc.* οἱ ἰατροί) φαρμάκῳ χολήν ('healers purge bitter bile with a bitter drug') as evidence of the controversy over different therapeutic systems and interprets this fragment through the lens of the explanation for pharmaceutical effectiveness in *Nature of Man* (esp. 5).

[35] This is especially true of *Airs, Waters, Places* and *Epidemics* 1 and 3, texts that are particularly concerned with the effect of the environment on human health. *Nature of Man* and *On the Sacred Disease* describe the affects of different seasons and types of weather on the humors in the body. The author of *Nature of Man* (cf. esp. 7) argues that all diseases arise from the effects of specific seasons on specific humors (thus, phlegm, the coldest humor, increases in winter, the coldest season); the author of *On the Sacred Disease* is also concerned with the influence of the weather, particularly moist, cold weather, on the brain, because he believes that epilepsy is caused by excessive phlegm (housed in the brain) going on the move.

[36] On the use of *metabolê* and other words for change in the Corpus, see Demont (1992).

not in general advocate drastic or wholesale change. Thus, the author of *Nature of Man* maintains that changes should be gradual, building up to more extreme measures if necessary (10); extreme changes can be detrimental to the patient's health. And in fact, those in the best of health can be most affected by change: *Aphorisms* 1.3 claims that because athletes are in peak physical condition, changes in their health can only be negative, inasmuch as there is really only one direction left for their health to go.

The author of *Regimen in Acute Diseases* criticizes an anonymous group of 'some healers' for prescribing major changes in regimen when trying to cure sick patients. He imagines their reasoning: perhaps they think that great changes in regimen are justified in response to the great changes effected by the disease (καὶ ἴσως τι καὶ εἰκὸς δοκεῖ αὐτοῖσιν εἶναι μεγάλης μεταβολῆς γινομένης τῷ σώματι μέγα τι κάρτα καὶ ἀντιμεταβάλλειν, 26: 'perhaps it seems likely to them that when a great change arises in the body that something very great also change in response'). But, he argues, such reasoning is faulty. He goes on to give numerous examples of situations where changes in regimen have a negative effect on health (28–35); consequently, if the healthy are harmed by unaccustomed diets, so much the more dangerous are such diets for the sick (31). The author is adamant that changes in regimen should be as slight as possible. Indeed, he notes that it may be detrimental to alter a customary regimen even when it is based on bad habits, since a change to unaccustomed habits may render the patient even worse:

> πολλὰ δ' ἄν τις ἠδελφισμένα τούτοισι τῶν ἐς κοιλίην καὶ ἄλλα εἴποι, ὡς εὐφόρως μὲν φέρουσι τὰ βρώματα, ἃ εἰθίδαται, ἢν καὶ μὴ ἀγαθὰ ᾖ· ὡσαύτως δὲ καὶ τὰ ποτά· δυσφόρως δὲ φέρουσι τὰ βρώματα, ἃ μὴ εἰθίδαται, κἢν μὴ κακὰ ᾖ· ὡσαύτως δὲ καὶ τὰ ποτά. (36 Joly)

> Someone might say as far as many other related issues involving the belly, how easily they bear the foods to which they are accustomed, even if they are not good; and it is also so with drink; but they bear with discomfort foods to which they are not accustomed, even if they are not bad; and it is also so with drinks.

Lest we think that such an attitude is confined only to this one author in some obscure corner of Greek intellectual life, we should note that there are parallels not only in medicine,[37] but also in other genres.

---

[37] The notion that moments of change are fraught with danger or that it is dangerous to change from what is customary turns up in many Hippocratic treatises: e.g., *Reg.*

Euripides himself provides evidence in fragments 201 and 282.[38] The context in which the Euripidean statements are made is unclear, but a similar line of reasoning appears in the clearer context of the debate between Nicias and Alcibiades over the merits of the Sicilian expedition, as represented by Thucydides.[39] Although Nicias claims to act as the healer of the state in advising against the expedition (6.14), Alcibiades cleverly turns this argument on its head (6.18.6–7). He maintains that Athens is now accustomed to war and the action of battle; thus, even if more war is to some extent unfortunate, altering the customary activity of the Athenians would create even greater suffering.

> παράπαν τε γιγνώσκω πόλιν μὴ ἀπράγμονα τάχιστ᾽ ἄν μοι δοκεῖν ἀπραγμο-
> σύνης μεταβολῇ διαφθαρῆναι, καὶ τῶν ἀνθρώπων ἀσφαλέστατα τούτους
> οἰκεῖν οἳ ἂν τοῖς παροῦσιν ἤθεσι καὶ νόμοις, ἢν καὶ χείρω ᾖ, ἥκιστα διαφό-
> ρως πολιτεύωσιν.

> And altogether I realize that a city that is not inactive would, it seems to me, very quickly be destroyed by a change to inactivity, and that among humans those live most securely who regulate their public life least differently from the established laws and customs, even if they are comparatively bad.

Similar arguments surface elsewhere in Thucydides, even if the medical metaphor is not so obvious. For example, there is Pericles' notorious statement about the nature of Athenian power: what you have is a tyranny, he says; while it may been wrong to acquire it, now that you have it, you must act in accordance with the responsibilities it entails

---

2.66, 3.68, *Aer.* 11, *Epid.* 3.17 (case 13); *Aph.* 1.20 (with the advice 'not to innovate' [μηδὲ νεωτεροποιεῖν] during or after a *krisis*), 2.49.

[38] Fr. 201 Nauck-Snell, from the *Antiope*, seems to have been part of the debate over lifestyles which took place between Amphion and Zethus: καὶ μὴν ὅσοι μὲν σαρκὸς εἰς εὐεξίαν / ἀσκοῦσι βίοτον, ἢν σφαλῶσι χρημάτων, / κακοὶ πολῖται· δεῖ γὰρ ἄνδρ᾽ εἰσθιμένον / ἀκόλαστον ἦθος γαστρὸς ἐν ταὐτῷ μένειν ('And indeed however many earn their livelihood / from the good condition of their flesh, if they lack money, / they are bad citizens; for a man accustomed to / reckless habits of eating must continue on the same course'). Fr. 282 Nauck-Snell, from the satyr play *Autolycus*, contains a long diatribe against athletes: they are basically useless to the state because they cannot withstand changes in regimen and must spend all their time concentrating on their health; so lines 8–9: ἔθη γὰρ οὐκ ἐθισθέντες καλὰ / σκληρῶς μεταλλάσσουσιν εἰς τἀμήχανον ('for if they do not customarily practice good habits, they change to uselessness') and lines 12–15: ἐμεμψάμην δὲ καὶ τὸν Ἑλλήνων νόμον, / οἳ τῶνδ᾽ ἕκατι σύλλογον ποιούμενοι / τιμῶσ᾽ ἀχρείους ἡδονὰς δαιτὸς χάριν ('But I blame also the custom of the Greeks, / who reasoning on account of these things, / honor useless pleasures for the sake of regimen').

[39] The parallel is noted and thoroughly analyzed in Jouanna (1980).

(2.63.2–3). In the same speech, Pericles confidently asserts, καὶ ἐγὼ μὲν ὁ αὐτός εἰμι (2.61.2: 'and I am the same [as I have always been]'), while criticizing his fellow Athenians for changing in response to the great change which has recently beset them (in this case, neatly enough for the medical parallel, the plague):

> ὑμεῖς δὲ μεταβάλλετε … διότι τὸ μὲν λυποῦν ἔχει ἤδη τὴν αἴσθησιν ἑκάστῳ, τῆς δὲ ὠφελίας ἄπεστιν ἔτι ἡ δήλωσις ἅπασι, καὶ μεταβολῆς μεγάλης, καὶ ταύτης ἐξ ὀλίγου, ἐμπεσούσης ταπεινὴ ὑμῶν ἡ διάνοια ἐγκαρτερεῖν ἃ ἔγνωτε. (2.61.2)

> But it is you who have changed … because grief [resulting from my policy] has already affected the perception of each person, whereas the clear nature of its benefit is absent for everyone, and since a great change—especially in a short time—has befallen, your state of mind is too low to persevere in what you have resolved.

Later, in the Mytilenean Debate, Cleon frequently echoes Pericles' statements (e.g., 3.38.1) as he argues that changing one's mind is a form of weakness.[40] Moreover, he maintains that a city benefits more from *nomoi akinêtoi* (undisturbed laws)—even if they are bad—than from excellent laws which are not enforced (3.37.3). Indeed, the issue of the potentially negative effects of change is clearly a 'hot topic' in the late fifth century.

Other Hippocratic authors seem to recognize the validity of the idea expressed in *Regimen in Acute Diseases*, but they also insist on the need to change diet in response to disease. The author of *On Ancient Medicine* points out that unaccustomed foods and changes in habit cause disease, but argues that changes in the diet are necessary for the sick, because their illness derives at least in part from what they have eaten (see, e.g., the discussion of cheese in ch. 20). Furthermore, as the author of *Regimen* argues, changes in nature result in disruptive changes within the body; thus, measures must be taken to counter these changes and to restore equilibrium (1.32.2). All the healers recognize that disease necessitates changes of some sort in order to restore health,[41] but a real tension develops in the Corpus when it comes to advising how

---

[40] On Cleon's echoing of Pericles, see Cairns (1982), who suggests that Thucydides includes this mimicry to the detriment of Cleon. But the words may also reflect an historical reality: cf. Hornblower (1991) *ad* 2.61.2.

[41] One solution is *metastasis*, a change of position, rather than a change in regimen or the use of *pharmaka*; cf., the change of environment recommended by the author of *Nature of Man* in the case of epidemic diseases (cited above, note 23).

such a change from sickness to health is to be effected. Stability is greatly valued, not only in medicine, but in Greek culture as a whole; inconstancy is not a virtue.

c. Apostasis

Apostasis is perhaps the hardest of these theoretical concepts to define, not because there are no reasonable English equivalents for the term nor because we cannot appreciate the importance of this notion of 'separation' or 'segregation' in Hippocratic thought.[42] The difficulty arises rather in understanding how and when *apostasies* occur, and, moreover, in distinguishing between *apostasis* as a cause of pain, *apostasis* as a sign of healing, and *apostasis* as a form of remedy. Langholf's discussion is particularly useful in describing the importance of *apostasis* to medical theory, though he, too, points to the difficulties in formulating an exact definition.[43] He cites the helpful description of *apostasies* in *Epidemics* 2.1.7:

> ἀποστάσιες ἢ διὰ φλεβῶν ἢ τόνων ἢ δι᾽ ὀστέων ἢ νεύρων ἢ δέρματος ἢ ἐκτροπέων ἑτέρων· χρησταὶ δὲ αἱ κάτω τῆς νούσου οἷον κιρσοὶ, ὀσφύος βάρεα, ἐκ τῶν ἄνω ἄρισται δὲ μάλιστα κάτω, καὶ αἱ κατωτάτω κοιλίης, καὶ προσωτάτω ἀπὸ τῆς νούσου, καὶ αἱ κατ᾽ ἔκρουν, οἷον αἷμα ἐκ ῥινέων, πῦον ἐξ ὠτὸς, πτύαλον, οὖρον, κατ᾽ ἔκρουν. οἷσι μὴ ταῦτα, ἀποστάσιες, οἷον ὀδόντες, ὀφθαλμοὶ, ῥὶς, ἱδρώς. ἀτὰρ καὶ τὰ ὑπὸ δέρμα ἐς τὸ ἔξω ἀριστάμενα φύματα, οἷον ταγγαὶ, καὶ τὰ ἐκπυοῦντα, οἷον ἕλκος, καὶ τὰ τοιαῦτα ἐξανθήματα, ἢ λόποι ἢ μάδησις τριχῶν, ἀλφοὶ, λέπραι, ἢ τὰ τοιαῦτα. ὅσα ἀποστάσιες μέν εἰσιν ἀθρόως ῥέψασαι, καὶ μὴ ἡμιρρόπως καὶ ὅσα ἄλλα εἴρηται κακὰ ἢν ἀναξίως τῆς περιβολῆς τῆς νούσου, οἷον τῇ Τημένεω ἀδελφιδῇ ἐκ νούσου ἰσχυρῆς ἐς δάκτυλον ἀπεστήριξεν, οὐχ ἱκανὸν δέξασθαι τὴν νοῦσον· ἐπαλινδρόμησεν, ἀπέθανεν.
>
> (Smith)

Apostases, through the blood vessels, the nerves, the bones, the tendons, the skin or other diversions. They are best when they go down from the disease, like varicose veins, heaviness of the loins. From the upper parts the best are the farthest below, those of the lowest intestine and farthest from the disease; also the ones that come by outflow, as blood from the nostrils, pus from the ear, expectoration, urine in its outflow.

---

[42] The writers express this notion of 'separation' with a variety of words; *apostasis* is the most common, but others include *apokrisis* and *diakrisis*. Both Langholf (1990) and di Benedetto (1968) use the term *apostasis* for the sake of convenience; di Benedetto stresses *apostasis* as one of the fundamental ideas in Hippocratic theories of remedy (4).

[43] Langholf (1990) 81–84.

> For those who lack these, expect apostases, for example, in teeth, eyes, nose, sweat. Also swellings under the skin which push out, for example scrofulous tumors and suppurations like ulcers, amd similar eruptions, or peeling skin, loss of hair, leprous skin, scaly skin or the like. All abscessions inclining in a mass, not gradually, and the others that have been described, are bad if inappropriate for the compass of the disease, as with Timenes' niece: from a strong disease it settled in her toe, which was not adequate to received the disease. It ran back up and she died. (trans. Smith)

Apostasis is linked with two other important concepts in the Hippocratic Corpus, *krisis* and *pepsis*. *Pepsis* (coction) seems to precede *apostasis*; it is the process by which substances are first broken down and then thickened in the body. After *pepsis*, the body is better able to expel bad substances (now in a form suitable for evacuation) through the various forms of *apostasis*. *Krisis* is the turning-point of a disease, the moment when the body gains the upper hand over its enemy, the attacking illness; in an incomplete *krisis*, the disease manages to fight its way back into contention. A *krisis* is often but not always accompanied by an *apostasis* (thus, the moment when the body manages literally to expel the disease), but it is difficult to say whether an *apostasis* causes a *krisis* or whether it is a sign that a *krisis* has occurred. Healers watch hopefully for nosebleeds, hemorrhoids, signs of excessive sweating, the onset of menstruation, and other forms of expulsion, all of which they believe may rid the body of the *materia peccans*. The body has the ability to perform the processes of *pepsis* and *apostasis* on its own, but healers may also try to help the sick body to perform them more successfully: thus, purges and klysters and emetics are directed at cleansing the body and removing the disease, usually through urine, feces, or vomit. Thus, *apostasis* is a particular kind of *katharsis*, a method by which the body is cleansed of disease.

Although complete expulsion is naturally to be preferred, even partial separation could be helpful. Healing mechanisms that may involve less than complete segregation are suggested in *Humors* 1, where the remedial strategies include *ekklisis* (deflection), *paroketeusis* (diversion) and *antispasis* (revulsion). Hence, Hippocratic writers report with seeming optimism both the relocation of disease into a less vulnerable part of a given patient's body and the diffusion of the disease across the body: the concentration of disease in one area is apparently more dangerous than its dispersal throughout the body. Thus, in a fuller description of the case of the niece of Timenes mentioned in the passage from *Epidemics* 2 quoted above, *Epidemics* 4.26 indicates that the transfer of a disease into the patient's big toe (together with diarrhea) is a potentially promising sign: unfortunately for the girl, the material ultimately came back to the main area of the body, and she died. This process is echoed in another case history from *Epidemics* 4.27, where the disease went to the feet and a crisis took place. In *Epidemics* 5.41, it first appears that even a diseased foot can be bad enough to cause death, but it should be noted that the patient also suffered from diarrhea before she died, indicating that the disease may have moved up into her cavity before becoming mortal. Other discussions, such as *Affections* 16, point out that even if the disease isn't expelled from the body, dispersal within the body can at least make the suffering more bearable, while a passage from *Diseases* 1 (20) maintains that if a small amount of diseased moisture disperses into the larger amount of healthy moisture present in the body, it becomes inconspicuous and painless, eventually becoming healthy once again. The treatise *Aphorisms* 2.46 maintains that if two pains occur at the same time in the body, but not in the same place, the stronger one obscures the weaker. As Helen King has remarked, 'the implications of this position for pain relief would suggest that you create a worse pain somewhere else to remove the one you started with.'[44] In the microcosm of the human body, bigger pains cancel out smaller ones. This seems to be the thinking behind some of the passages in *Epidemics*, such as 2.5.2, 2.5.9 and 2.6.25, where problems with the mouth or coughing or in the upper areas generally are relieved by the development of strong pain in the lower parts of the body. Such a remedy may also be hinted at in 2.5.4, in a passage concerning trauma to the head, where the author argues that the head, the chest, the hypochondrium and the hip cannot all be in pain at the same time: hence, perhaps the healer should try to shift the pain to these other areas in order to clear up the pain in the head.

However, a tension also exists regarding the notion of separation. *Krasis* or *mixis*, the balanced blending of bodily substances, is essential to health. The movement of a particular substance into a state of separation, the collection of a substance into one place, isolated from its normal situation and separated from the balanced *krasis* of the rest of the body (and thus disrupting that balance)—this is dangerous, causing pain, disorder, disease. Yet once this occurs, the body must

---

[44] King (1998) 122.

work to disperse the substance from its point of collection,[45] to expel the separated substance, to rid itself of the noxious excess. Thus, *apostasis* necessitates further *apostasis*, and at the same time, the body must recover from this expulsion in order to restore itself again to a balanced whole.

d. Malthakia *and* ischys

As Herodotus' account of Democedes demonstrates (3.130), Greek healers had long prided themselves on the gentleness of their methods; they had deliberately moved away from cutting and burning except in the most extreme cases. Many of the treatises recommend the use of 'soft' foods, drugs, or purges, while criticizing the potentially negative effects of 'strong' remedies. For example, Ann Hanson has discussed the changing attitude of Hippocratic healers with regard to the traditional remedies represented in the gynecological treatises, specifically in *Diseases of Women*. She shows how author C (as Grensemann identified the author of the latest stratum he discerned in these treatises) criticizes the use of harsh pessaries (involving cantharid beetles, among other things) to treat uterine inflammation; author C argues that such harsh methods will only make the condition worse.[46] *Affections* 61 maintains that foods eaten by the healthy person are too strong when eaten by the sick, and advises removing the 'strength' of the food before administering it to the patient. The authors of *Regimen* and *Regimen in Acute Diseases* recommend different treatments for different types of patients, but both authors advise the use of foods that are soft and easily digestible when dealing with sick patients; they certainly are opposed to extreme or harsh types of food in any case.

As with all generalizations about the Hippocratic Corpus, this one must also admit significant modifications. The author of *Airs, Waters, Places* praises light, sparkling, sweet-smelling water that flows from the east—but he states this is not best for every type of constitution (7.9–11). Someone who is healthy can drink anything, he says, but the hardest and saltiest water is appropriate for the person who has a stomach that is soft, moist and full of phlegm (7.13). While the gynecological

---

[45] Other terms for this dispersal are *apolysis* and *dialysis*, both of which express a process of dissolution.
[46] Hanson (1991) 80–81.

treatises generally advocate soft remedies and soft foods as a matter of principle, they in fact give a wide range of cures. For example, Hanson's article discusses the use of succussion in childbirth, which could involve shaking the woman up and down on a ladder.[47] *Diseases of Women* 2.121 states that if a women is strong, give her strong medicine; if she is weak, then weak medicine is appropriate. *Barren Women* 217 (= *Superfetation* 29) advises proceeding from weaker drugs to stronger ones, although this passage also warns that strong drugs can be dangerous. *Places in Man* presents another mixed picture, advocating the application of strong drugs to strong people and weak drugs to weak people (27). Furthermore, this author's general theory on therapeutics includes the advice in chapter 34 (repeated in 45) that weak diseases can admit strong remedies, but that strong or unidentifiable disease should be treated only with weak drugs—no doubt the body under attack by a strong disease could not withstand the onslaught of harsh medication as well. The *Aphorisms* too offer some pithy advice about degrees of treatment in medicine: *Aphorisms* 1.7 and 1.8 recommend the lightest possible diets for those in the throes of an acute disease; 1.9 suggests that in the race between disease, healer and patient, the healer should consider whether the patient is strong enough to bear a particular diet: ξυντεκμαίρεσθαι δὲ χρὴ καὶ τὸν νοσέοντα, εἰ ἐξαρκέσει τῇ διαίτῃ πρὸς τὴν ἀκμὴν τῆς νούσου, καὶ πότερον ἐκεῖνος ἀπαυδήσει πρότερον, καὶ οὐκ ἐξαρκέσει τῇ διαίτῃ, ἢ ἡ νοῦσος πρότερον ἀπαυδήσει καὶ ἀμβλυνεῖται ('it is necessary to examine the patient, if he is strong enough for the diet at the height of the disease, [and to consider] whether the patient will be exhausted first and not be strong enough for the diet, or the disease will be blunted and exhausted first'). *Aphorisms* 7.87 assesses the severity of basic types of treatment in three stages: ὁκόσα φάρμακα οὐκ ἰῆται, σίδηρος ἰῆται· ὅσα σίδηρος οὐκ ἰῆται, πῦρ ἰῆται· ὅσα δὲ πῦρ οὐκ ἰῆται, ταῦτα χρὴ νομίζειν ἀνίατα ('what drugs do not cure, the knife will; what the knife does not cure, cautery will; what cautery does not cure must be considered incurable'). Here it is surely implied that cautery must be used only as a last resort, and that one should begin with less severe forms of treatment. However, *Aphorisms* 1.6 points out that the most extreme cases require the most extreme remedies. It seems that there are times when the harsher methods in the healers' repertoire must be put into use.

---

[47] Hanson (1991) 91–92.

CHAPTER SIX

FINDING THE CAUSE AND FINDING THE CURE: FOUR EURIPIDEAN PLAYS

a. Orestes: *No way out*

The myth of the Tantalids provides fertile ground for tragic explorations of violence, suffering, disease and remedy. Euripides begins the *Orestes* with a prologue in which Electra describes how the *symphora* (disaster) and the *nosos* of Tantalus have been perpetuated throughout the generations of his descendants. Tantalus begins the story: the *makarios* (blessed) man who has the honor of feasting with the gods gets into difficulty because of his *nosos*—an *akolaston glôssan* (unbridled tongue), says Electra (10); she does not tell the story we know from Pindar of the ghastly banquet in which Tantalus tried to serve his son to the divinities. Nor does she relate the specific horrors perpetrated by Tantalus' descendants. Indeed, Euripides makes his Electra insist on elaborate praeteritio throughout the first twenty-three lines of the prologue; Electra names the 'criminals' but not their crimes.[1] Only the details of Orestes' case are provided. Yet Orestes is linked with his ancestor Tantalus by the theme of *nosos* (10 and 34).[2] And the stories of the gen-

---

[1] Unless perhaps at line 15, which Murray, Biehl and West include, but which di Benedetto, Willink and Diggle delete. I am inclined to agree with the arguments of the latter three, who maintain that Electra hints throughout the prologue, but does not give specifics. However, the case can only be made on the contextual argument; the objections to the line itself are not strong. Dunn (1996) 163–164 connects Electra's halting speech with the theme of unbridled speech and repressive silence that runs throughout the play. Neither speech nor silence works as a strategy for Orestes and Electra: moreover, by speaking out boldly, they show that they have inherited the disease of their ancestor.

[2] On the figure of Tantalus as a negative motif recurring implicitly and explicitly throughout the play, see O'Brien (1988). Among other points, he argues that there is an important link between the frequent threat of stoning directed at Orestes and Electra in the play and the tradition (found in Alcman, Archilochus, Alcaeus and Pindar) that Tantalus was threatened by an overhanging stone as punishment. Kyriakou (1998) argues against O'Brien that the play does not stress the negative aspects of Tantalus' myth; she prefers to see Pelops as the truly problematic ancestor in the play. Tantalus

erations intervening between Orestes and his notorious ancestor are revealed gradually, in the agones and in the choral odes of the play: after the insolent activity of Tantalus, each generation, confronted with hideous acts of kin-killing and child-eating or child-sacrifice, attempts to counter this violence with reciprocal acts of violence. It is clear that Orestes, too, has caught this disease; he, too, by killing his mother, becomes a participant in the family tradition and suffers from the inherited curse.

In the literary versions of this myth, immortal figures play a very active role in this final generation just as they did in the case of Tantalus himself—now, it is no wife, brother, or child who attacks, but rather the Furies who pursue Orestes and Apollo who eventually arrives to defend him. There are no opposing family members left, it seems, who might carry on the tradition of opposition; hence, the gods must take over. In *Orestes*, Euripides imitates a mythical situation also found in Aeschylus' *Oresteia*, but Euripides introduces new and additional violence into the story. The Aeschylean Orestes seeks and finds some refuge from the advocacy of Apollo and then true remedy from Athena and the Athenian court of justice. The trilogy finds a new remedy for the problems in the House: justice is removed from a cycle of kin-violence and placed under the protection of a jury. The Orestes of the *Eumenides* has no interest in taking vengeance on Helen, or abusing the name of his uncle Menelaus, or rebuking Apollo in his absence; like his Euripidean counterpart, he seeks peace, freedom from madness, and a future, but he does not think to find such things by means of additional violence.

In the *Eumenides*, mortal and immortal figures come together to put an end to the cycle of violence that has for so many generations possessed the house of the Tantalids. Orestes is purified, the case is closed with a verdict which acquits him of wrong-doing. Moreover, the Furies are transformed into the Semnai, the Kindly Ones (1041), and their inherent capacities are redirected:[3] they are now to bestow peace and fertility upon the land, as long as no citizen engages in

---

does not have much significance in the *Oresteia*—Aeschylus concentrates rather on Atreus and Thyestes as progenitors of the quarrel.

[3] Aeschylus associates the Furies with the local Athenian goddesses, the Semnai, and may have been the first to do so. 'Eumenides,' by contrast, seems to have been a common (and euphemistic) alternative name for the Furies in Athens and elsewhere; the term does not occur in the *Oresteia*, but was used in post-Aeschylean references to the play. Cf. Sommerstein's edition of *Eumenides*, pp. 10–12.

blood feuds or vendettas. A court has been established which is to treat cases of homicide, even those occurring among family members. In the future, there will be no need, and no right, for a son to act as Orestes has.[4] Euripides gives us a rather different version of the story, and the remedies that he presents are conflicting and inconclusive.

Euripides notoriously introduces the anachronism of a pre-existing homicide court at Argos into the dramatic situation of the *Orestes*.[5] Tyndareus argues that Orestes had no need to take justice into his own hands; Clytemnestra had indeed deserved death, but that sentence could have been, and indeed ought to have been, carried out by a court rather than by an individual family member. Furthermore, we are told in the opening scenes of the play that Orestes labors under two different threats of death, death from the madness and the attendant exhaustion which he suffers due to the pursuit of the Furies, and death by stoning to be imposed by the Argives as punishment for the matricide. As the play progresses, the violence worsens; the threat of madness and the Furies seems muted in the presence of the terrifying measures which Orestes, Pylades and Electra are willing to undertake—murder, hostage-taking, conflagration. The mortals of the play come to such a state of irresolvable conflict that only the intervention of Apollo is able to settle it, and only by divine fiat. The play suggests that human institutions of justice are rendered powerless in the face of madness, greed, jealousy, and cowardice—the gods alone can put a stop to human evils and they can only do so by the drastic measure of direct intervention.

Yet we learn this lesson (if this is indeed the lesson to be learned) only at the end of a play in which the human characters have repeat-

---

[4] This is perhaps a naïve reading of Aeschylus' intentions and Aeschylus' trilogy, which scholars such as Goldhill (1986) have argued does not end on an unequivocally positive note. But the contrast between the two young heroes is strong, and I maintain that the contrast between the Euripidean and Aeschylean accounts is in general strong as well.

[5] See discussion in Porter (1994) 126–128. While the anachronism of the homicide court has provoked much discussion (for a review, see Porter [1994] 126 n. 89 and 127 n. 95), the strangeness of Orestes' own trial scene at the Argive assembly has been overlooked. Why should Orestes himself be tried at an assembly and not prosecuted in a homicide court if such a court was available in the case of his mother? As many scholars have argued, the messenger's report of the assembly reflects contemporary Athenian political events; replacing the formal trial of Orestes before the Areopagus with a 'trial' of Orestes at an assembly may be Euripides' way not only of contrasting his hero with that of Aeschylus in the *Oresteia* but also of remarking upon the political climate in Athens at the time. See Hall (1993) 266–268.

edly tried to remedy the situation for themselves. Electra first prescribes sleep for the troubled Orestes; Orestes later prescribes sleep for his suffering sister. Both are hopeful that Menelaus will help them. When it turns out that he is reluctant to do so, Orestes tries another approach: he attempts to justify his actions to the assembly and so win acquittal for himself. When this course of action fails, Pylades proposes a new tactic: win the respect and gratitude of the population by killing Helen, the root cause of so much destruction. Electra even sees a way to force the hand of Menelaus: she proposes that they take Hermione hostage and threaten to kill her if Menelaus refuses to help them. In the confusion of the final scene of the play, the three conspirators appear ready to burn down the palace and to kill Hermione just when Menelaus appears to have capitulated to their demands. It is in the midst of such imminent and senseless destruction that Apollo makes his entrance, just in time to set the narrative back onto its traditional mythic course.

One may of course analyze all these schemes and twists of plot in terms of dramatic structure and technique. But if we look more closely at the language with which characters propose and discuss these actions, we can hardly help but notice the frequency with which medical themes turn up. To suggest that Euripides wove such motifs into the fabric of his *Orestes* is perhaps hardly startling in light of Smith's work on the importance of disease imagery in the play.[6] Other scholars, too, have illuminated different functions of the disease motif: Jouanna and Boulter have discussed the savagery (*agria*) that characterizes both the disease in the play and the play itself;[7] Parry has considered the disease theme in the context of his analysis of the play as a quest for salvation.[8] Garzya has drawn comparisons between Orestes' symptoms and descriptions of mental disturbances in the Hippocratic Corpus.[9] More recently, Hoessly has remarked upon the similarities between symptoms of Orestes' disease and those found in *Diseases of Young Girls*, on the one hand, and a disease styled the 'thick disease' described in *Internal Affections* (48), on the other.[10] Yet none of these scholars has attempted

---

[6] Smith (1967).

[7] Boulter (1962); Jouanna (1988).

[8] Parry (1969).

[9] Garzya (1997), with special reference to *On the Sacred Disease*, *Epidemics* 3.17 (11) and 15 and *Diseases* 2.72.

[10] Hoessly (2001) 137–140. She reminds us that the author of *Diseases of Young Girls* indicates that men can suffer from the same symptoms he describes, even though they are more typical of women.

an analysis which examines the disease theme specifically in terms of therapeutics.[11] In fact, in their discussions of remedial action, the characters of the play touch upon major types of remedial theory that we find in the medical authors. As we shall see, the characters variously consider soft versus harsh methods, allopathic and homeopathic cures, and *metabolê* as opposed to invariability. Furthermore, the play seems to explore the problematic relationship between exterior and interior causes discussed in the medical writers. For Orestes' own case involves, on the one hand, the external influence of Apollo and the attacks of the Furies and, on the other, the innate disordered *physis* of his family and the troubled *synesis*, the interior 'awareness,' on which he also blames his madness.

Electra and Orestes

Let us begin by examining the notions of remedy operative in the early scenes of the play. In the prologue, having catalogued the history of various family horrors, Electra describes the immediate plight from which she and Orestes suffer: Orestes lies on stage, sick, exhausted by the attacks of the Furies; moreover, brother and sister are both threatened with death sentences. The opening lines of the play stress the severity of the suffering that afflicts the *physis* of all humankind:

> Οὐκ ἔστιν οὐδὲν δεινὸν ὧδ᾽ εἰπεῖν ἔπος
> οὐδὲ πάθος οὐδὲ ξυμφορὰ θεήλατος
> ἧς οὐκ ἂν ἄραιτ᾽ ἄχθος ἀνθρώπου φύσις.   (1–3)

> There is no word so terrible to say,
> nor suffering nor god-sent disaster,
> whose pain the nature of man could not bear.

We should note that Electra has three categories here, a terrible word, suffering, and disaster, and that the first two are not qualified as 'god-driven.'[12] Her family exemplifies the human capacity for enduring all

---

[11] Although Hoessly (2001) does suggest that perhaps the ending of the play, in which Orestes is ordered to marry Hermione, contains a therapeutic idea derived from *Diseases of Young Girls*: just as young women should have sexual relations with men to relieve the madness that besets them, so too should Orestes sleep with Hermione to relieve his 'misogynen Verfolgungswahn' (143).

[12] I understand the syntax thus: the ὧδε is modifying δεῖνον, which in turn is qualifying ἔπος; εἰπεῖν is epexegetical with ἔπος. Ἔπος, πάθος and σύμφορα are all in the nominative. The words are arranged in a tricolon, capped by the σύμφορα θεήλατος. (There are manuscripts which have *symphora* in the accusative, in which

three types. In the narrative that follows, Electra hints at the particulars
of these complex forces of causality at work. Although she admits that
crimes have been committed by her ancestors, she asserts that divine
forces are to blame for the current suffering—Apollo has improp-
erly commanded Orestes to kill Clytemnestra, the Furies are making
Orestes sick. Yet Electra has no expectation of divine help at this junc-
ture; rather, she announces that the siblings have one hope of safety:
Menelaus (52–53). However, the history of intra-familial betrayal and
corruption which she has just narrated runs counter to such hopes for
help from kin—or so at least members of the audience may conclude.

Euripides' stagecraft serves to reinforce this lack of confidence. Electra ends her speech by informing us that she is waiting anxiously for
Menelaus to arrive. Tragic conventions lead us to expect that in fact
the next person to appear on stage will be none other than the man
himself.[13] Instead, it is Helen who makes an appearance, a rather foolish and timid Helen. Her rather inappropriate request that Electra perform libations on her behalf at Clytemnestra's tomb is the occasion for
yet another pronouncement from Electra on *physis*: ὦ φύσις, ἐν ἀνθρώ-
ποισιν ὡς μέγ' εἶ κακόν (126: 'o nature, how great an evil you are for
men'). She goes on to explain that Helen has proved herself 'the same
woman of old' (ἡ πάλαι γυνή, 129)—her nature has not been altered by
circumstance. From a literary stand-point, Helen seems almost less than
at least some of her former selves:[14] she is not the sad and resourceful
woman from Euripides' own *Helen*, nor does she have the skill in *pharmaka* with which the Helen of the *Odyssey* removes the feelings of pain
and sorrow. In this play, however, Helen's behavior serves to remind us
that neither side of Electra's family has an irreproachable history, while
Electra's own commentary reminds us of the belief found in even the
most optimistic medical writers: diseases can be cured, but the fundamental nature of a person cannot be altered.

---

case *pathos* and *epos* would be accusative, too. But the nominative has good manuscript
authority.) Willink's notes on this passage are slightly misleading because he seems to
translate the passage one way (commentary *ad* 1–3) and explain the syntax another
(commentary *ad* 1–2).

[13] Cf. Willink *ad* 71–125. He adduces Taplin's discussion of Euripides' 'penchant for
"surprise" entrance-technique' (*Stagecraft of Aeschylus*, 10–11).

[14] Willink likens her to the Helen of the *Iliad*, with some qualifications. He argues
that she is motivated in this scene by *aidôs* and *philia*. However, the situation surely
points up the contrast between the Helen of the *Iliad*, shown respect in general by the
Trojans and certainly an object of some awe, and this Helen, sneaking about, afraid to
be seen, fearful for her life.

Electra herself can do nothing to cure Orestes of his madness, but she is a loyal, steadfast nurse. She speaks to Helen of her *prosedria* (attendance at bedside, 92), which Orestes later mentions as a source of possible danger to Electra's own health (304–305). Orestes is in fact a difficult patient: as Electra tells us in the prologue, in periods of sanity, he has been lying in bed, unwashed, not eating and weeping; by contrast, when madness seizes him, it gives him the strength to leap about like a colt. When the kind but noisy chorus enters, she desperately tries to prevent it from waking her brother from the sweet gift of sleep.[15] The chorus and Electra engage in a rather extended exchange regarding Orestes' condition. This dialogue adds little to the audience's knowledge about Orestes' sickness (already discussed by Helen and Electra). Rather, it emphasizes both the importance of Orestes' sleep and the dim prognosis for his recovery or his future. Orestes, Electra states and the chorus agree, will surely die:

Χόρος. θρόει τίς κακῶν τελευτὰ μένει.
Ἠλέκτρα. θανεῖν ⟨θανεῖν⟩, τί δ᾽ ἄλλο;
    οὐδὲ γὰρ πόθον ἔχει βορᾶς.
Χόρος. πρόδηλος ἄρ᾽ ὁ πότμος.   (187–190)

Chorus. Tell what end of evils remains.
Electra. Death, death, what else?
    For he has no desire for food.
Chorus. So then the outcome is clear.

Sleep is clearly considered to be helpful and restorative here, but it is equally clear that Electra does not wish her brother to awaken for other reasons as well—because she can do nothing to help him and because she fears that madness will overtake him once again. In other tragic sleep scenes, the wakeful characters speculate about what may happen if the sleeper wakes up, but the results of the actual awakening prove benign (at least for the other characters). The standard pattern seems to be crisis, followed by restorative sleep, then followed by sober awakening and sorrowful denouement (thus, death of the tragic hero eventually results in *Aias* and *Trachiniae*, whereas the hero lives on in *Heracles* and *Philoctetes*).[16] Moreover, the scene reverses the events in the

---

[15] Of course, the noise of the chorus is unavoidable, linked as it is to the convention of the loud anapaestic parodos. There may also be some metatheatrical play here (typical of Euripides): if the chorus does not enter, the play cannot be staged—which might, given the horrible events to follow, be better for all concerned (I owe this point to Ann Hanson).

[16] On sleep scene patterns, see Jouanna (1983); on therapeutic scenes more generally,

play's dramatic predecessor, the *Eumenides*, where it is the Furies who sleep, worn out by their pursuit of Orestes. Here, the crisis precipitating the sleep occurs before the time of the play and madness follows it. Although Electra speaks of sleep as a *charis* (gift, 159), it becomes clear that sleep will neither cure nor rescue Orestes; it may permit him temporary relief from mental distress, but it removes neither the onset of madness nor the threat of death.

The chorus asks fearfully whether Orestes is in fact not asleep, but dead (208–210). Orestes himself answers that question by waking up immediately to address sleep as ἐπίκουρος νόσου ('helper against disease,' 211). Sleep brings him forgetfulness, a gift which madness (that is, presumably, loss of reason) ironically does not. However, his condition has hardly improved. Electra touches him with soothing strokes and tries to ease his sickness with gentle attention. The fractious patient is too weak to lift himself or to brush his hair out of his eyes. Reinforcing Electra's observations in the prologue,[17] he explains that when the disease releases him, he becomes weak, unable to control his limbs and to stand: ὅταν ἀνῇ νόσος / μανίας, ἄναρθρός εἰμι κἀσθενῶ μέλη (227–228). The disease is still in charge here, releasing and seizing the patient at will. Sleep has brought forgetfulness, but not recovery. In the battle against disease, this patient is losing. Orestes also remarks upon the *aporia* of the sick (δυσάρεστον οἱ νοσοῦντες ἀπορίας ὕπο, 232: 'the sick are hard to please because of their desperate situation'), which recalls Electra's earlier statement that the house of the unfortunate is 'a resourceless thing' (ἄπορον χρῆμα, 70). Once again, Euripides uses the disease motif to underscore the desperation of the youngest generation of this family: not only do they lack the resources to cure Orestes' madness, but they literally have 'no way out' of the situation— the house, the boundaries, the roads are all guarded, Menelaus will soon claim he has no power to help, Pylades has been disowned by his father, the people of Argos are against them, led by an angry Tiresias and an enemy, Oiax, inherited from their father.[18] Medical theory

---

see Kosak (1999), with discussion of the significance of this therapy scene (110–114), arguing that it reveals a negative slant on Orestes' character because of his lack of independence.

[17] χλανιδίων δ' ἔσω / κρυφθείς, ὅταν μὲν σῶμα κουφισθῇ νόσου / ἔμφρων δακρύει ...(42–44: 'but hidden inside his cloak, whenever his body is relieved of the disease, he weeps in his self-awareness').

[18] In contrast to tragic Thebes, where the stuff of tragedy is in-born and seemingly ineradicable, Argos is a place where, according to Saïd (1993), 'tragic action always

stresses the importance of expelling the sick material. But Orestes cannot escape; thus, he and his disease, inseparable from one another, can only implode.

But we will return to that issue later. After all, Electra does not give up easily on her brother, for all her gloomy predictions. She urges her brother to stand up, reasoning that μεταβολὴ πάντων γλυκύ (234: 'change of everything is sweet'). This is indeed an interesting pronouncement, especially since it is made in a therapeutic context. As we have seen, *metabolê* is an important principle in Hippocratic therapeutics. Electra, however, gives an excessive version of the *metabolê* principle, in which the merits of change are 'sweet' in all circumstances. Given the cautious approach to *metabolê* in the therapeutics advocated by the medical writers, Electra's statement is of dubious legitimacy. Her words may encourage her brother, but they can only inspire suspicion in the audience. And indeed, the play proceeds to complicate the merits of Electra's suggested therapeutics immediately. Only moments later, when a fit of madness overtakes Orestes, Electra is aghast at the change: ταχὺς δὲ μετέθου λύσσαν, ἄρτι σωφρονῶν (254: 'swiftly you have changed to a state of madness, when just now you were sane'). Moreover, in a choral song and monody later in the play (960–1012, especially 979–1012), a tension is developed between the need for change and the possibility of danger inherent in change. The antistrophe mourns the loss of fortune in the once blessed (ἐπὶ μακαρίοις, 972) house of the Tantalids, ending with a more general reflection on constant exchange of various troubles which comprise human life:

> ἕτερα δ' ἕτερον ἀμείβεται
> πήματ' ἐν χρόνῳ μακρῷ·
> βροτῶν δ' ὁ πᾶς ἀστάθμητος αἰών.   (979–981)

> But every pain is exchanged for another one
> in the long course of time;
> and the whole life of mortals is unstable.

The monody retells the story of the house, focusing on the misdeeds of Pelops and his sons, Atreus and Thyestes.[19] In particular, it stresses the terrifying *metabolê* of the sun which occurred in response to the deeds of Atreus and Thyestes:

---

comes ... from the outside' (174) and which one attempts either to leave or to enter: as she puts it, 'Argos is but a starting or a stopping place' (168). She notes how Euripides places great stress on the inability of Orestes to leave Argos in the *Orestes* (185).

[19] On the significance of Pelops in the play, see Kyriakou (1998), who argues

ὅθεν Ἔρις τό τε πτερωτὸν
ἁλίου μετέβαλεν ἅρμα,
τὰν πρὸς ἑσπέραν κέλευθον
οὐρανοῦ, προσαρμόσασα χιονόπωλον Ἀῶ,
ἑπταπόρου τε δράμημα Πελειάδος
εἰς ὁδὸν ἄλλαν [Ζεὺς μεταβάλλει].   (1001–1006 West)[20]

Hence Conflict turned the sun's winged car about
to the westward sky-course, having yoked on
the snowy steeds of Dawn
and turned the running of seven-track Pleiad
onto another path.

But even this drastic change in nature has not managed to change
the situation for Electra's family; indeed, they continue to exchange
not just *pêmata*, but death: τῶν δ᾽ ἔτ᾽ ἀμείβει θανάτους θανάτων (1007:
'from these deaths there came yet more deaths'). So entrenched are
their ways that the laws of nature alter rather than the nature of
the family. The play thus asserts the need to alter the characteristic
behavior of the Tantalids, while at the same time giving frightening
examples of change, change which is characterized by the abnormal or
the unnatural: the madness of Orestes and the retrograde motion of the
sun. Euripides' changes to the story, which add two murder attempts to
Orestes' slate, also contribute to the theme, reminding the audience
that it is not change in and of itself which is important, but rather the
direction and purpose of the change.

Orestes does not choose to modify or contradict his sister's statement
about change, however. He agrees to her suggestion that he change
positions with the words: μάλιστα· δόξαν γὰρ τόδ᾽ ὑγιείας ἔχει. / κρεῖσσον δὲ τὸ δοκεῖν, κἂν ἀληθείας ἀπῇ (235–236: 'certainly: for this has the
appearance of health; for the appearance is stronger, even if it is far
from truth'). At the end of the scene, as Electra departs to get some
rest, she advises her brother to stay in bed, concluding: κἂν μὴ νοσῇ
γὰρ ἀλλὰ δοξάζῃ νοσεῖν, κάματος βροτοῖσιν ἀπορία τε γίγνεται (314–315:
'for even if you are not sick, but only appear to be sick, [even in this

---

that Pelops is stressed at this point in part to help us interpret the actions of Menelaus:
Menelaus is repeating the bad behavior of his ancestor Pelops by refusing to perform
an act of *charis* in compensation for the benefits he has received from Agamemnon and
Orestes.

    [20] West has attempted to solve the crux at 1003–1004 (which remains as such in
Diggle's text: οὐρανοῦ † προσαρμόσας / μονόπωλον ἐς Ἀῶ †, /ἑπταπόρου τε δραμήματα
Πλειάδος / εἰς ὁδὸν ἄλλαν Ζεὺς μεταβάλλει ...).

situation] suffering and despair exist for mortals'). Thus, Orestes asserts the strength of positive thinking and action in the face of illness, and Electra later responds with a statement about the ability of negative thinking and action to create illness. Yet only the negative version of this appearance/reality dichotomy proves tenable in this scene, for an attack of madness overtakes Orestes soon after his pronouncement. It is possible to appear less than you are, but not more.[21] Actual sickness and apparent sickness lead to the same situation—*aporia*—whereas apparent health is no substitute for real health and no match, certainly, for madness. Remedy is not to be found in *to dokein* (appearance).[22] Moreover, the famous bow of Apollo[23] with which Orestes is to defend himself against the attacks of the Furies fails to ward them off completely; it is now the sixth day that he must contend with their onset. And Electra's suggestions, consisting basically of sleep or *metabolê*, fail to heal her brother; moreover, her constant attendance at her brother's bedside results only in the danger of becoming ill herself, as Orestes recognizes. Both siblings exhibit a blend of optimism and pessimism in this scene: they hope for help from Menelaus and they believe in the possibility of change; but at the same time, they admit despair, anger, and *aporia*. They no longer expect assistance from the gods and yet recognize that their own human resources are scarce indeed.

Orestes and Menelaus

The next scene presents us at last with the arrival of Menelaus and the meeting between uncle and nephew. As I discussed in my analysis of the play in Part I, the scene represents Menelaus as a healing figure, but one who is unsuccessful. Here, I shall focus on the issues of remedy that arise in the scene. As noted above, after an initial discussion of Orestes' appearance and symptoms, we learn first that Orestes' disease results

---

[21] Unless of course a goddess makes you appear extraordinary (as Athena will often do for her favorites). But heroes on their own can only make themselves look less spectacular; thus, e.g., the disguises of Odysseus and Telephus as beggars, Achilles as a girl (less spectacular in the Greek world-view).

[22] However, Padel (1992: 187–188) suggests that this equivalence between seeming and reality is an essential feature of the Erinyes themselves and also an 'important truth' asserted by the play.

[23] Potentially an issue of *to dokein* in and of itself! The problem of the reality or unreality of the bow (see discussion in Willink *ad* 268–274) is not one that I can address here, but an imaginary bow would serve to reinforce the issue of being and seeming introduced by Orestes and Electra.

from his realization that he has done 'terrible things' (ἡ σύνεσις, ὅτι σύνοιδα δείν' εἰργασμένος, 396: 'self-awareness, that I know that I have done terrible things'). This explanation is, as I have said in my earlier discussion, unintelligible to Menelaus, and so Orestes proceeds to give a more customary set of causal factors, grief and madness. We next learn more specifics about the madness: when it started, where it first occurred, what form it takes. Orestes then claims to have an *anaphora* for his *symphora*, a release for his disaster (414)—not suicide, but Apollo, who ordered him to kill Clytemnestra. Since Apollo caused him to take on this suffering, he should be responsible for removing it. Menelaus is not impressed, arguing that the god acted foolishly (417) and moreover is a long time in coming to the rescue (419). When Orestes counters that the gods take time to act as part of their divine nature (μέλλει· τὸ θεῖον δ' ἐστὶ τοιοῦτον φύσει, 420: 'there is delay: for the divine are naturally that way'), Menelaus points out that the Erinyes managed to arrive almost immediately (423)—delay is not a characteristic of all divinities. The conversation reaches a turning point when Orestes admits that his act of vengeance has not yet done him any good:

Μενελάος. πατρὸς δὲ δή τι σ' ὠφελεῖ τιμωρία;
Ὀρέστης. οὔπω· τὸ μέλλον δ' ἴσον ἀπραξίᾳ λέγω.   (425–426)

Menelaus. But does the avenging of your father help you in any way?
Orestes. Not yet: and I claim that [constant] delaying is equivalent to no action at all.

Indeed, the healing god is nowhere in evidence and the remedy which he prescribed has resulted in yet more disaster for the house of Atreus.

The two surviving males of that house now turn from the intimate concerns of Orestes' disease to an analysis of the social conditions (τὰ πρὸς πόλιν, 427). Once again, Menelaus seeks out the particulars, this time of persons and their positions; he inquires as to the seriousness of the situation, learning that death by stoning is the most probable outcome. His one suggestion—flight—is rejected as impossible by Orestes, who explains that there are guards on all the boundaries (444). At last, as mentioned in my earlier discussion, Menelaus gives his diagnosis—and prognosis: ὦ μέλεος, ἥκεις συμφορᾶς ἐς τοὔσχατον (447: 'o wretched one, you have come to the last point of disaster'). The wealthy and fortunate Menelaus clearly feels that there is nothing he can do, indeed, nothing to be done, to improve the situation; because the prognosis for Orestes is death, Menelaus can devise no strategy for cure.

The arrival of Tyndareus shifts the focus of the scene to a closer consideration of Orestes' past actions in terms of justice and injustice. Tyndareus' arguments leave Menelaus shaken; the agon conducted by Tyndareus and Orestes has impressed upon him the isolation of Orestes and Electra and the unpopularity of their position. After Tyndareus' angry departure, Orestes manages to persuade his uncle to hear him out and resumes his efforts to obtain his help. His arguments are certainly rather unusual. Moreover, he presents his case in terms that are strikingly homeopathic: 'I have committed injustice,' he says; 'now I require injustice from you in order to balance my wrong-doing' (ἀδι- κῶ· λαβεῖν χρή μ' ἀντὶ τοῦδε τοῦ κακοῦ / ἀδικόν τι παρὰ σοῦ, 646–647). Orestes stresses the blood which Agamemnon and Menelaus share, the similarities of their family situations, and yet the gross imbalance between the respective prices which the brothers have paid for the Trojan expedition and thereby the honor of the family. Euripides clarifies the medical context informing Orestes' reasoning in the words with which he describes Agamemnon's actions in Troy: he went there unjustly (ἀδίκως, 648) in order to heal injustice (ἀδικίαν ... ἰώμενος, 650). Menelaus' act of injustice will likewise re-establish equilibrium by healing Orestes' act of injustice against his mother.

The argument Euripides presents here is no doubt meant to be shocking. Moreover, it is a variation on a similar motif found in Aeschylus fr. 349, μὴ κακοῖς ἰῶ κακά ('lest I heal evils with evils'). Radt's edition of the Aeschylus fragments includes a lengthy list of passages in both Greek and Latin literature which echo the sentiments of this fragment.[24] It is important to note that in all of these passages, the homeopathic method of remedy is presented as something to be avoided, whether because it is considered dangerous, foolish, or ineffective. Yet Orestes in his plea to Menelaus argues against this piece of wisdom, insisting boldly that injustice can heal injustice.

---

[24] These include Hdt. 3.53.4, μὴ τῷ κακῷ τὸ κακὸν ἰῶ ('so that I may not heal trouble with trouble'); Soph. *Aias* 362, μὴ κακὸν κακῷ διδοὺς ἄκος πλέον τὸ πῆμα τῆς ἀτῆς τίθει ('do not, in adding a bad pain to a bad one, make the bane of the disaster worse'); Soph. fr. 77, ἐνταῦθα μέντοι πάντα τἀνθρώπων νοσεῖ / κακοῖς ὅταν θέλωσιν ἰᾶσθαι κακά ('hence indeed everything among humans is sick whenever they wish to heal evils with evils'); Eur. *Bac.* 839, κακοῖς θηρᾶν κακά ('to hunt down evils with evils'); and Thuc. 5.65.2, τῶν πρεσβυτέρων τις Ἄγιδι ἐπεβόησεν ... ὅτι διανοεῖται κακὸν κακῷ ἰᾶσθαι ('One of the elders shouted out to Agis ... that he was considering healing trouble with trouble').

Although Orestes never specifies exactly what type of unjust action
he envisions, Menelaus clearly understands it to be some type of armed
intervention. In his reply, Menelaus cautiously rejects such forceful
methods. Scholars have often argued that Euripides' version of Menelaus in this play is meant to be a thoroughly unsympathetic character
(at least until the final scene, where he pleads for the life of his innocent daughter). And certainly the cautiousness (*eulabeia*) that characterizes his stance has potentially negative political overtones.[25] Yet it is also
true that his rejection of the homeopathic remedy proposed by Orestes
and his advocacy of gentle methods would place him in the company of
many Hippocratic healers. Inasmuch as Menelaus has exclaimed over
the extreme nature of Orestes' suffering (447), his recommendation of
eulabeia and *malthakia* certainly contradicts the advice in *Aphorisms* 1.6:
ἐς δὲ τὰ ἔσχατα νουσήματα αἱ ἔσχαται θεραπεῖαι ἐς ἀκριβείην, κράτισται
('the most extreme cases require the most extreme treatments'). On the
other hand, Menelaus could reason with the author of *Places in Man*
that Orestes is too weak to sustain stronger methods. Menelaus also
offers his own weak position as an explanation of his inability to act on
Orestes' behalf; he can only suggest that by allowing events to run their
course, Orestes may eventually gain what he wants. The question of
intervention is a major one in Hippocratic treatises. Von Staden's article on incurability in the Hippocratic Corpus includes analysis of physicians' attitudes towards intervention. His study reveals a firm belief that
action taken by a healer in the early stages of disease has a much better
chance of success; moreover, errors made by the healer in these early
stages 'tend to be reversible or "easier to remedy".'[26] The frequent references to the time elapsed since Orestes has fallen ill indicate that the
disease is no longer in its infancy. The most common periodicities in
the Corpus comprise four, seven or fourteen days.[27] Orestes has been
sick for six days—perhaps it is too dangerous to intervene at this point.
However, von Staden also shows that despite the frequency with which
diseases in the Corpus are described as incurable, the healers nevertheless seem to believe that in most cases 'there is no such thing as

---

[25] For *eulabeia* and Menelaus, see 699, 743, with Willink *ad* 682–716, 696–703, and
further discussion of the term in Willink (1990) 183–185.
[26] Von Staden (1990) 87.
[27] See discussion in my earlier analysis of *Orestes* in Part I, pp. 87–88.

intrinsic incurability.'[28] The good healer always stands a chance in his fight against the disease.

Thus, Menelaus would seem to have faced both criticism and praise were he to be judged by a panel of Hippocratic physicians. Orestes' suggestion that he treat *adikia* with *adikia* would certainly not meet with much approval (at least on moral or theoretical grounds), yet Menelaus' unwillingness to act in any significant way would meet with harsher judgment. His advocacy of soft methods seems reasonable (although he fails to undertake even these), but again, some might suggest that the severity of the situation requires stronger medicine. Menelaus does have one other set of factors which might argue in his favor: as von Staden points out, although most authors in the Corpus seem to believe that no disease is intrinsically incurable, there are three important exceptions. For the rationalist healers do assert, first, that defects in the *physis* of the individual can occur, against which the healer has no chance; second, that defects exist *kata genos* (inherited) or *ek genês* (from birth)—often closely linked, of course, with defects arising *physei* (by nature)—which are again unassailable by medical arts; and third, that healthy people can suffer accidents so severe that healers can do nothing.[29] Certainly, Orestes' disease seems to fit into the second of these categories, if not also the first. Many healers would argue that it is wrong and foolish to attempt a cure in such cases, since the inevitable failure of the healer's *technê* would result in loss of respect for the healer and for the profession as a whole.[30] From this perspective, Menelaus' position appears perfectly intelligible: no Greek man wishes to lose respect, and Orestes' case certainly appears quite hopeless.

Orestes and Pylades (and Electra again)

When Menelaus departs, Orestes dismisses his promises as equivalent to nothing.[31] Orestes claims that 'the house of Agamemnon is clean gone' (τὰ δ' Ἀγαμέμνονος φροῦδα, 720–721; the adjective recalls for us Orestes' earlier description of his body as φροῦδος, 390). No longer

---

[28] Von Staden (1990) 91.
[29] Von Staden (1990) 93–95.
[30] Cf., e.g., *Ars* (esp. ch. 8) and *Prog.* 1.
[31] And, indeed, the report of Menelaus' inaction at the assembly bears out Orestes' reaction.

has he any hope of escaping death. Nevertheless, upon the arrival of his friend, kinsman, and co-conspirator Pylades, he begins to seek out fresh alternatives. As has happened repeatedly thus far in the play, the gravity of the situation is again rehearsed (Electra in prologue; Electra to Helen; Electra to chorus; Electra and Orestes; Orestes to Menelaus; Orestes to Pylades). In spite of the new arrivals and the fact that we have heard over 700 lines of the play, the basic problem has not altered, nor has it come any closer to resolution. Yet one has to admire Orestes for his tenacity. Spurred on by the encouragement of his friend, he decides to attempt persuasion. Inasmuch as his previous efforts at persuasion have failed to move even those who are blood-relatives (*homaimoi*, 806), it is perhaps not surprising that he does not succeed at the assembly either. Indeed, the only persons willing to support Orestes are some country folk at the assembly, the chorus of women, Pylades, and Electra. It appears that Orestes is too late in his attempt to use softer methods to solve situations. Rather than beginning with a softer approach and moving to a harsher one as necessary, Orestes has begun with the harshest method of all. He has already resorted to violence in killing his mother; he has demonstrated an unyielding lack of repentance for what he has done (although he regrets that he is now suffering the consequences); he has sought violent action on his behalf from Menelaus. Now at last he will try the softer approach advocated by his uncle. What Orestes did not grant to his mother, he will now grant himself: the process of justice (crude as the process reported by the messenger seems to be).

The exchanges we have thus far witnessed between Orestes and his *philoi*, his friends and relatives both true and false, have shown us two possible approaches to remedy. Electra, powerless to help with regard to the political situation, concerns herself with the effects of madness on Orestes; she sits by her brother, tends to him, worries about him, and tries to prevent further damage by urging him to rest, but she cannot cure him. Menelaus also has no remedy for the madness; he recommends caution and gentleness in dealing with the community. Now it is Pylades' turn. Cut off by his father and exiled from his homeland, he too lacks the ability to cure Orestes of madness and the resources either to help him escape or to improve his chances with the assembly. However, he agrees with Orestes' own plan of action and is more than willing to help carry it out. He promises to tend to Orestes should the madness seize him during the assembly. Moreover, Pylades shrugs off the possibility that he may become infected by coming into physical contact with the polluted man (792–794).[32] Indeed, Pylades is determined to suffer with his friend, insisting not only on his loyalty, but also on his participation in every aspect of the plot—both dramatic and mythical. If Pylades has ever been overlooked or downplayed in other dramatic versions of the Orestes myth, he seems determined to make sure that he will not be forgotten here.

When Orestes returns from assembly now in actual fact sentenced to death, he is resigned to his fate. Electra is more resistant—it takes some time and persuasion before she is willing to yield to the death sentence. Pylades insists that he, too, will take part in the death scene which is to come. Yet now the action begins to move from 'softer' methods to 'harsher' ones, from persuasion to violence. For Pylades also suggests additional action: if they have to die, he says, they should at least find some way to make Menelaus 'suffer too' (συνδυστύχῃ, 1099). Why does Euripides introduce this new twist into the plot? Why does Orestes cheerfully embrace it? What good will it do the three conspirators, doomed to death as they are? The traditional Greek ethic of helping friends and harming enemies is certainly at work—Menelaus has been removed from the circle of *philoi* and placed into the enemy camp. But, as I have indicated in my discussion of the concept of *apostasis*, some ideas from the Hippocratic Corpus can also help us. As noted above, *Aphorisms* 2.46 states that a stronger pain developing in another part of the body will cancel out a weaker one. *Nature of Man* 11.1 suggests venesection behind the knees in order to reduce pains in the back. *Affections* 16 argues that if phlegm or bile gather together, they each have the power to dominate, producing pain in the site where they have assembled; if dispersed, however, 'they are weaker in any part of the body in which they appear.' Although the Hippocratics do not try to spread disease, many seem to agree with the author of *Affections* that disease and pain are caused by the excessive concentration of a substance in a particular area; dispersal (*apolysis, dialysis*) will reduce pain. Perhaps this notion is suggestive of a common way of thinking

---

[32] Critics often compare Theseus' statement in *Heracles* that he does not fear contracting pollution through touching Heracles since οὐδεὶς ἀλάστωρ τοῖς φίλοις ἐκ τῶν φίλων (1234: 'no avenging spirit comes to friends from friends'). But we should observe an important distinction here: Theseus denies the contagion of pollution, whereas Pylades says he does not care about it. Pylades is eager to suffer with and even die with his friend—he never denies that Orestes' 'disease' may be contagious, and in fact he seems quite willing to contract it.

in the fifth century: the concentration of suffering on one individual is
more painful than the shared suffering of many.

Pylades suggests another *phonos*, the murder of Helen. The chorus
has already lamented the traditional 'homeopathic' exchange of *phonos*
for *phonos* in the house of the Tantalids (816–817);[33] it is clear that
the previous murders have never remedied matters in the family. But
Pylades foresees additional benefits to the plan. He predicts positive
reactions from a population overjoyed at Helen's death; he maintains
that Orestes will no longer be known as *mêtrophontês*, the matricide
(1140), but rather as the *Helenês ... phoneus*, the slayer of Helen (1142).
The language at this point is noteworthy:

> ὁ μητροφόντης δ' οὐ καλῇ ταύτην κτανών,
> ἀλλ' ἀπολιπὼν τοῦτ' ἐπὶ τὸ βελτίον πέσῃ,
> Ἑλένης λεγόμενος τῆς πολυκτόνου φονεύς.   (1140–1142)

> Having killed this woman [Helen] you will not be called the matricide,
> but having left this name behind you will take a turn for the better,
> being called the murderer of much-killing Helen.

Pylades predicts that Orestes, 'leaving behind' the name *mêtrophontês*,
will 'take a turn for the better,' as West translates the phrase ἐπὶ τὸ βελ-
τίον πέσῃ. This translation aptly brings out the medical tone of Pylades'
words, for *epi to beltion* is indeed a medical expression, occurring only
very rarely in any of the other prose or poetical works of the fifth century.[34] By contrast, it appears often in the medical writers in contexts
describing improvements in health. Pylades thus believes that Orestes'
condition will improve with a change in his reputation—and indeed,
were Orestes not known as the *mêtrophontês*, his prospects for life, liberty
and freedom from madness would be much greater. However, the lesson of Orestes' family history has been rehearsed enough times already

---

[33] Diggle (following arguments made by Willink *ad loc.*) prints πόνῳ πόνος in place of
the φόνῳ φόνος transmitted by the manuscripts. That these *ponoi* include acts of murder
is made clear by the phrase δι' αἵματος in 817.

[34] There is one non-medical use in fifth-century prose (Thuc. 7.50.3), no other
instances in tragedy, and three occurrences in Aristophanes (*Nub.* 589, 594, *Eccl.* 475).
Plato uses the expression six times, Aristotle, three. Even in later authors, it appears
more frequently in medical literature than in any other genre, with the exception of
some Christian writers. The expression occurs eleven times in the Hippocratic Corpus. The comparable expression ἐπὶ τὸ ἄμεινον occurs four times in the Hippocratic
Corpus, twice in Herodotus, and nowhere else in extant fifth-century literature. It most
commonly occurs in combination with the verbs συμφέρειν, ἐπιδιδόναι, and μεταβάλ-
λειν.

in the play to demonstrate that additional acts of violence do not cancel out or reverse previous ones; rather, they only perpetuate the family disease. Furthermore, the name *phoneus*, even if it is modified as *Helênês phoneus*, is not much of a substitute. This is no cure, but at best a desperate attempt to stabilize the disease.

Orestes accepts Pylades' plan with enthusiasm, believing that vengeance on Menelaus is a good start; moreover, should unexpected safety (ἄελπτος ... σωτηρία, 1173) for the killers of Helen result as well, this would mean true happiness (εὐτυχοῖμεν ἄν, 1172). But it is up to Electra to propose the crowning touch of violence, which she maintains will yield certain *sôtêria* (1178, now stripped of the qualifying *aelptos*). As Electra unfolds her plan to take Hermione hostage, the play's recurrent medical motif resurfaces explicitly. Orestes, not yet understanding the purpose of Electra's proposal, inquires: τίνος τόδ᾽ εἶπας φάρμακον τρισσοῖς φίλοις; (1190: 'for what purpose do you speak of this *pharmakon* for three friends?'). Electra explains the function of the suggested *pharmakon*: the threat of yet another murder will accomplish their rescue by 'softening' (μαλάξειν) the *splanchnon* of Menelaus (1201). Now, Menelaus' advocacy of soft methods is not only turned against him, but in fact reversed. Violent, forceful methods will soften the enemy, as opposed to soft methods which might blunt the opponent's strength. Indeed, it will not even be that difficult, says Electra, since Menelaus is neither bold nor strong by nature (1201–1202). The softness of Menelaus himself has been implied throughout the play, beginning with the *habrosynê* (softness) by which he is characterized upon his first entrance.[35] Softness is a physical attribute of women—men are supposed to be hard and firm.[36] Thus, Electra's plan is intended to soften the soft man even further, to disrupt his bodily equilibrium, and to reduce him to the status of a woman. Her prescription is at once homeopathic and allopathic: homeopathic, in that it prescribes the additional murder of Hermione to cure any trouble caused by the murder of Helen; allopathic, in that the harsh murder of Hermione (or rather, the threat of murder) will soften Menelaus' *splanchnon*. By prescribing murder, she will save her brother, herself and Pylades; at the same time, her plan is intended to weaken Menelaus so that he will be forced to use his strength on their behalf. Electra's suggested course of therapy is complex: it uses Hermione and Helen as drugs which are

---

[35] See Willink *ad* 348–351.
[36] For a medical reflection of this wide-spread view, cf., e.g., *Glands* 16.

to operate on Menelaus; he, in turn, is to become the means by which Orestes, Pylades and Electra are cured.

Thus, it seems that at last a *pharmakon* has been found. After a hasty set of prayers to invoke the help of Agamemnon, the three *philoi* hurry off to perform their respective parts in the plan. But despite their elaborate schemes and the glee with which they carry out these additions to the traditional plot, it becomes clear that they are not so certain of success after all. Once the murder of Helen has been attempted and the capture of Hermione has taken place, we hear the details of the story from a Phrygian slave who escapes from the palace. Orestes soon emerges in pursuit of this unarmed slave, in order to catch him before he can tell the Argives what has happened. The womanly Menelaus can come, says Orestes (1532);[37] he is certainly no threat. But Orestes is concerned about unfavorable popular reaction (1529–1530, 1533–1534), no longer so confident about that joyous response to the news of Helen's death which Pylades envisioned (in part, perhaps, because Helen has disappeared and Orestes does not know exactly what has happened to her).

In the final confrontation with Menelaus, the logic of the conspirators' plan becomes confused. Whatever the textual problems (and there are many), the course of events seems established:[38] Orestes first maintains that he doesn't look for rescue, but rather intends to burn down the palace (1594); then he demands that Menelaus induce the city to rescind the death sentence (1610–1611); then, having exacted an admission of defeat from Menelaus (ἔχεις με, 1617: 'you've got me'), he tells Electra to set the house afire anyway (1618), and seems prepared to go ahead with the murder of Hermione. In the midst of this chaos, which threatens to put an end to the entire family, Apollo makes his entrance, re-routes the action, and resolves the crisis. He orders them to dissolve their quarrels (1679) and to honor Peace (1682–1683). The mortals assent (although Orestes does so with a measure of hesitation, worrying at 1686–1689 that this may be an *alastôr*'s trick) and seem ready to live happily ever after.[39] If only medical problems were so easily remedied.

---

[37] A clear echo of the Archilochean poem on the general (114 West) and a further indication of Menelaus' reputation for *habrosynê*.

[38] Even though Willink proposes some significant rearrangements of the text in this scene, he does not alter the general sequence of action described here. His 'BCAD' rearrangement seems the most satisfactory solution.

[39] The ending of the play has occasioned much comment from critics, who point to

b. Heracles: *Politics, plagues and the patient*

The *Heracles* is a play riddled with illness. Stasis, old age, madness, pollution—all these are in some way characterized as diseases. Yet the play has resisted the attempts of scholars to explain the relationship between all these parts. Direct links between the stasis in the city and the madness of Heracles are hard to find; furthermore, the elaborate set-up of the political situation in Thebes seems to go for naught, as all mention of the issue vanishes in the second part of the play. However, it seems to me that the play does offer a consideration of potentially different ways by which disease might infiltrate a society and its leaders; disease in *Heracles* stems variously from contagion, from the environment, and from the gods.

There have been many attempts to illuminate the unity of the two halves of the *Heracles*.[40] Parallels have been noted, themes discussed, motifs traced. Moreover, the play presents striking reversals: the usurper Lycus' pre-emptive strike against Heracles' family mirrors Hera's vicious act of revenge (at last put into action now that Heracles has completed his labors); similarly, Heracles kills the very wife and children whom he had rescued in the first part of the play. Many critics have struggled to explain Euripides' treatment of the myth, in which Heracles kills his wife (Megara in this play) and children after his completion of the labors. Other versions of the myth usually situate the slaughter of the children at a time early in Heracles' career, and do not mention the killing of Megara at all.[41] Wilamowitz maintained that Heracles shows signs of megalomania in the first part of the play which anticipate the full-fledged madness described in the messenger speech.[42] Burnett focused not so much on Heracles proper, but rather on the

---

its forced quality. See the contribution of Dunn (1996), esp. 170–171, who shows how Apollo's solution does not help the audience make up its mind about the tenor of the play: has it been a tragedy or a comedy? The ending imposed by Apollo, argues Dunn, 'confirms this impasse' (171), thus contributing again to the theme of *aporia* that dominates the play. By contrast, Sourvinou-Inwood (2003: 400) argues that the ending suggests that there is after all a divine order, unknowable to humans, but asserted by the fact that Apollo does rescue Orestes in the end, confirming that it was right for Orestes (and humans generally) to obey the gods.

[40] For some overviews of the scholarship on 'unity,' see Bond, pp. xvii–xxi and Michelini (1987) 231–233.

[41] For the 'traditional' order of events and the myth of Heracles' madness, see Bond pp. xxvi–xxx.

[42] Wilamowitz *ad* 562–582.

blasphemy against Zeus exhibited by Heracles' mortal father Amphitryon and Megara; in her view, Heracles' actions are a punishment for
this sacrilege.[43] While I do not claim that the disease theme solves all
the interpretive problems of the play, I nevertheless believe that a consideration of this theme can help us to understand the role of the first
part of the play in setting up the second. Thus, I would suggest that the
stasis at Thebes acts as an environmental factor, and one that comes
to infect Heracles as well as the citizens of Thebes.[44] Just as Euripides turns from considering the political situation in Thebes in the first
half of the play to confront the tragedy within Heracles' family in the
second, so, too, does disease transfer from the larger entity of the city
to the body of Heracles himself. Through both dramatic situation and
imagery, the play suggests that the external disorder of political stasis materializes as the internal disorder of personal madness. On the
other hand, the play presents a very clear instance of divinely caused
disease, and moreover introduces the issue of contagion, particularly
in the scene between Heracles and Theseus. Furthermore, the play
explores not only issues of disease causation, but also aspects of doc-
toring and remedy. Both halves of the play consider various forms of
remedy, from the cures provided by nature itself to the particular skills
of one man, from the omnipotence of Zeus to the healing powers of
a well-ordered community. The well-ordered city-state of Athens, personified by its leader Theseus, manages to rescue Heracles, but the fate
of Thebes remains unknown: the chorus' last words speak only of their
grief at having lost 'the greatest of *philoi*' (1428).

Stasis

The internal disorder of the city is stressed throughout the first half
of the play, beginning with Amphitryon's description in the prologue.
In contrast to the happy and unified processions by which the Thebans
had celebrated the marriage of Heracles and Megara some years before
(9–12), the city now suffers from factionalism: it is literally 'sick with
stasis' (34). Heracles' departure for his series of world-taming labors
seems to have left the city vulnerable to inner strife and to attacks from

---

[43] Burnett (1971) 159–172.
[44] For further discussion of the influence of 'environment' in Euripides, see Diller
(1960).

outsiders. This has in turn led to the precarious situation in which Amphitryon, Megara and the three sons of Heracles find themselves: with the city in disarray, the tyrant Lycus has seized the opportunity to kill them off. Any hope of help from old friends seems to be rendered vain by this combination of factionalism and tyranny. In the absence of Heracles, the inner turmoil at Thebes appears to have no solution. Turmoil elsewhere in Greece (i.e., the monsters and terrors described in the lengthy choral ode running from 348–441) has met its match in Heracles the tamer and cleanser himself.[45] In the course of the play, we learn that he has even managed to tame the Underworld to a degree, by removing Cerberus from its gates. He will soon reveal the power to return from the dead, a power granted to very few mortals indeed. But both the recent and the more distant history of Thebes related by Amphitryon reveals several generations of political strife, from the earlier Lycus, to Amphion and Zethus, to the new Lycus who has overtaken the sick city.

The background of political turmoil is stressed throughout the play. Indeed, the word stasis explicitly occurs more times in *Heracles* than in any other extant tragedy. In lines 272–273, as the aged members of the chorus express their outrage over the treatment of Heracles' family and bemoan their own inability to provide redress, they complain that the city, 'sick with stasis,' is not thinking well; otherwise, it would never have accepted Lycus as ruler. Again, at 542–543, as Heracles seeks information about the terrible plight of his family, he asks whether Lycus has achieved power by force of arms or through some sickness of the land. Megara gives a one-word reply: stasis. Bond suggests the alternatives given by Heracles are really the same thing, implying that Lycus' arrival precipitated the stasis in Thebes.[46] But the phenomena of stasis and the rise of a tyrant, although related, are distinctly different in the Greek mind. They are in fact two stages in the process of change in constitutional form (*metabolê politeias*), and, significantly, stasis comes first. Stasis refers to interior power struggles between pre-existing factions within a city; these factions may be supported by external agencies, as often happened in the actual situation of the Peloponnesian War. According to Greek theories of constitutional change, stasis weakens the state and gives rise to tyrants. The actual conditions that lead to civic breakdown

---

[45] For Heracles as tamer, see 20 and 852; as cleanser, see 225.
[46] Bond *ad* 543.

vary only slightly among sixth- and fifth-century authors. Solon, writing in a pre-democratic period, attributes the rise of stasis to a cluster of moral and economic factors: in poem 4 West, he describes a process whereby wealth leads to *koros* (satiety) among the ruling aristocracy (7–11). *Koros* results in hybristic and unlawful behavior (12–14), causing dissatisfaction among the lower classes (23–25). Clashes between the various factions lead ultimately to the emergence of a single individual, the tyrant, as ruler.[47] Solon's reforms aimed at finding common ground in the middle of the extremes of wealth and poverty, aristocracy and masses, with the ultimate goal of forestalling the drastic changes in constitutional form which were perceived as extremely harmful to society (cf., e.g., poem 36 West). Yet despite Solon's efforts on behalf of Athens, the tyrant Peisistratus rose to power not long after Solon made his attempts at polis reform.[48]

In the fifth century, Protagoras[49] located the cause of political instability once again in the loss of moral restraints—in this case, *aidôs* and *dikê*, which Protagoras felt were essential to *eukosmia*, the proper and stable order of any well-functioning polis. A state must continue to encourage and preserve the values of *aidôs* and *dikê*; otherwise, it will deteriorate into a more primitive condition, one in which tyrants flourish.[50] Fifth-century thinkers stressed that endurance is an important criterion for a good constitution and that the lawgiver's most important task is to construct a constitution which will resist alteration. Thus, Theramenes argued that modified oligarchy (e.g., the rule of the Five Thousand, which, however, did not endure) provided a middle course between the extremes of arrogant tyranny and radical democracy.[51] Others, such as Thrasymachus (cf. DK85 B1), stressed the need for *homonoia* (like-mindedness, shared communal values) as a stabilizing fac-

---

[47] Solon does not speak of tyranny in poem 4, but in poem 9, which describes a similar process of political breakdown, he speaks of the demos as subject to the power of one ruler since the city has been destroyed by the 'great men.' In his study of Greek theories of political change, Ryffel (1949: 15–21) argued that Solon understood stasis to lead to tyranny.

[48] Herodotus makes it clear that Peisistratus rose to power as a tyrant when the city of Athens was already suffering from civil strife (1.59).

[49] As transmitted to us by Plato in *Protagoras*, esp. 320d–351e.

[50] Note that at line 557 Megara stresses Lycus' lack of *aidôs* when she describes to Heracles the current situation in Thebes, while at the same time attributing the general cause of their personal difficulties to stasis in the city at large.

[51] Thucydides 8.97.1.

tor: in so far as different laws and customs obtain in different communities, citizens within those communities must all be willing and committed to follow the same social principles; otherwise, social strife and civic breakdown will occur. In the historians Herodotus and Thucydides, both economic and moral factors play a role in the development of stasis. Herodotus stresses the role of pride and ambition (*philotimia*),[52] Thucydides, the combination of *philotimia* and *pleonexia* (greed).[53] It is not only greedy and hybristic behavior among the wealthy that contributes to stasis in the societies described by the historians, but also similar passions stirred up among the poorer classes.

As this brief sketch has indicated, the general outlines of stasis theory remain fairly consistent in Greek thought throughout the sixth and fifth centuries. Whatever the actual form of constitution, whether it be monarchy (rare among the Greeks themselves during the period when the stasis theories are being developed), oligarchy, democracy, or variations of these forms, stasis threatens to arise when the ruling entity turns away from traditional values of restraint or loses respect for the laws. Hybristic and immoral behavior leads to breakdown, which then leads to tyrannical rule, itself characterized as rule without restraint. Stability (*eukosmia*) is to be achieved through shared communal values (*homonoia*), either through the good order (*eunomia*) that traditionally characterized the Spartan system, or the order based on equality (*isonomia*) to which Athens aspired.

Lycus' legitimate connections to Thebes are denied from the very beginning; it is rather his outsider status that is stressed (Καδμεῖος οὐκ ὢν ἀλλ᾽ ἀπ᾽ Εὐβοίας μολών, 32: 'not being a Cadmeian but coming from Euboea').[54] Thus, Megara's answer to Heracles at line 543 supports what the chorus said earlier: the city was infected with stasis and did not think well; it brought such a tyrant on itself because of internal discord. The final mention of stasis in the play, at lines 588–592, gives a

---

[52] It should be noted that Herodotus also uses the notion of sickness in combination with stasis, when he describes Miletus as a city νοσήσασα … στάσι at 5.28.1. The word *philotimia* occurs only once in Herodotus (3.53), but the idea that people take on more than they should out of ambition (rather than merely out of greed, though this may play an unspoken role) is very common: for example, the proverbially wealthy Croesus in Book 1 surely does not attack the Persians merely because he seeks greater riches, but because he desires more power and fame (and also is destined for a fall because of the sins of his ancestor, Gyges, according to 1.91).

[53] Cf. analysis in Macleod (1979) and the extensive discussion of Price (2001).

[54] Reiterated by the chorus at 256: … οὐ Καδμεῖος ὤν ('not being a Cadmeian').

fuller description of the discord in Thebes than any of the previous
references. In this passage, Amphitryon warns Heracles against the
greedy men supporting Lycus who have set up stasis and destroyed the
city:[55]

> πολλοὺς πένητας, ὀλβίους δὲ τῷ λόγῳ
> δοκοῦντας εἶναι συμμάχους ἄναξ ἔχει,
> οἳ στάσιν ἔθηκαν καὶ διώλεσαν πόλιν
> ἐφ᾽ ἁρπαγαῖσι τῶν πέλας, τὰ δ᾽ ἐν δόμοις
> δαπάναισι φροῦδα διαφυγόνθ᾽ ὑπ᾽ ἀργίας.

> Many poor men—although claiming to be wealthy—
> the master has as allies,
> who have set up a stasis and destroyed the city
> through pillaging of their neighbors, since the wealth in their own
>   houses
> is clean gone from lavish expenditures and dissipated by laziness.

While the individual Lycus has killed the previous king Creon and
become tyrant, it is the Theban followers of Lycus who have destroyed
the city. Amphitryon's statement reinforces the chorus' earlier remarks.
Amphitryon and the chorus are clearly scornful of Lycus, attacking
him for *dysgeneia* (base birth) among other things, but they criticize
the *philoi* of Heracles and indeed all the citizens of Thebes for their
betrayal; Lycus is after all an outsider and he only acts the way any
tyrant would,[56] whereas the descendants of the Spartoi have given in
once again to civil discord and are destroying their city and benefactors such as Heracles.[57] These portraits of the political situation in
Thebes fit into the general picture of stasis as it was painted by Euripides' contemporaries.[58] Certainly the disordered thinking mentioned by

---

[55] Amphitryon's remarks point to a group traditionally attacked for causing trouble
in the state: Bond *ad loc.* gives as parallels Plato *Rep.* 555d, Plut. *Aristides* 13, Lysias 25.11.

[56] See Connor (1977).

[57] A tension appears to exist between the pride in their Cadmeian heritage expressed
by the chorus of Theban elders and shame over the behavior of the citizens of Thebes;
such tension results in the frequent shifts in blame as the chorus (and Megara and
Amphitryon) sometimes directs its criticism at Lycus, sometimes at the Thebans.

[58] Tragedy rarely presents a political situation that exactly parallels a contemporary
Greek constitutional set-up: it was no doubt difficult to fit together the hereditary
kingships of mythology with the democratic system of Athens or even the oligarchic
systems of other Greek states. Yet this does not mean that tragedy will not have
exploited contemporary political tensions or theoretical discussions. Cf. Scodel (1982),
where she argues that the chorus in the second stasimon of *OT* is expressing fear of
stasis, and that within the context of traditional Theban monarchy, Sophocles is using
the chain of hybris→stasis→tyranny. Scodel also cites *Heracles* as an example of Greek

the chorus finds a parallel in Thucydides' description of the stasis at Corcyra, where *philotimia* and *pleonexia* lead to factionalism and ultimately to disrespect for all traditional law and order. The chaos at Corcyra is exemplified for Thucydides by the breaches of sanctuary laws, the intra-familial killings and the lack of respect for oaths (3.81.5; 3.83.2). The similarities Thucydides suggests between the effects of the plague at Athens and of the stasis at Corcyra have not gone unnoticed.[59] Euripides states directly that stasis is a disease which infects cities; its symptoms, as seen in *Heracles*, are disorder, lack of respect for legitimate rulers and customs, breaking of sanctuary laws, and the rise of tyranny. The similarities between Thucydides and Euripides indicate, I think, that the image of stasis as a disease or plague was not an uncommon one in the late fifth century.[60] Perhaps even more disturbing for our understanding of *Heracles* are not only the ways in which the situation in mythical Thebes parallels Thucydides' account of the stasis at Corcyra, but also the fact that Heracles himself becomes a participant in the typical course of events. After all, Thucydides also describes how fathers killed their sons at Corcyra (3.81.5). Indeed, Heracles' arrival and his subsequent actions seem not to slow the course of disaster at Thebes but rather to intensify it.

As much as Euripides' portrait of Thebes reflects Greek descriptions of political stasis, it also provides an interesting twist on the Presocratic Alcmaeon of Croton's explanation of health and disease, which is of course rife with political metaphors:

---

thinking on the rise of tyrants: tyrants take advantage of an unstable political situation, they do not cause it (218). On tragedy and politics, see also Saïd (1998).

[59] See Connor (1984) 242–245.

[60] Cf. also the passage in Herodotus mentioned above (note 123), the references to Plato (*Soph.* 228a, *Rep.* 470c, 556e) cited by Bond in his commentary on *Heracles*, 542, and Ar. *Vesp.* 650–651: χαλεπὸν μὲν ... / ἰάσασθαι νόσον ἀρχαίον ἐν τῇ πόλει ἐντετοκυῖαν ('it is difficult to cure an ancient disease born in the city'). Although the city's disease in *Wasps* does not seem to be stasis, it appears to be a 'political' disease of some kind. However, it is unclear from Bdelycleon's speech exactly what the disease is meant to be: jury-duty is characterized as a disease in the beginning of the play, but in the speech here, Bdelycleon criticizes the stupidity of the people who allow themselves to be deceived by those in power and are thereby cheated out of their share in the profits of empire. For further discussion of stasis as a disease, see Kosak (2000); for a discussion of medical imagery, including stasis, as it is applied to Greek cities, see Brock (2000); for another example of extended thematic use of disease imagery in a political arena, see Kallett (1999).

τῆς μὲν ὑγιείας εἶναι συνεκτικὴν τὴν ἰσονομίαν τῶν δυνάμεων, ὑγροῦ, ξη-
ροῦ, ψυχροῦ, θερμοῦ, πικροῦ, γλυκέος καὶ τῶν λοιπῶν, τὴν δ' ἐν αὐτοῖς μο-
ναρχίαν νόσου ποιητικήν· ... τὴν ὑγείαν τὴν σύμμετρον τῶν ποιῶν κρᾶσιν.

(DK24 B4)

The balance [equality of rights] of forces [in the body]—wet, dry, cold,
hot, bitter, sweet, etc.—maintains health, whereas monarchy [the domination of one force] among them is productive of disease. Health is the
balanced mixture of these [forces].

For Alcmaeon, balance (*summetria*), mixing (*krasis*), and the equality of
rights (*isonomia*) of different bodily substances meant health, whereas the
separation of bodily substances and the domination (*monarchia*) of any
one of them caused disease. The *Heracles* actualizes these metaphors in
its portrait of a city that, in its disintegration into factionalism, threatens
to destroy the family of one of its greatest benefactors. Indeed, the situation into which Heracles arrives is characterized by *taragmos*, another
concept that makes its most prominent Euripidean appearance in this
play. In political discourse, *taragmos* (and its relatives ταραχή, τάραξις,
and ταράττω) goes beyond stasis in its implications of disaster: although
violent and terrible, stasis at least can take place in an organized fash-
ion, carried out by different groups with specific agenda, but *taragmos*
implies total disruption and lack of direction—in short, anarchy. Thus,
Thucydides uses the concept to describe the utter breakdown of *nomoi*
that occurred during the plague in Athens (νόμοι τε πάντες ξυνεταρά-
χθησαν, 2.52.4: 'all the laws were completely disrupted'),[61] and to portray the chaos and tragedy experienced by the Athenians during the
Sicilian campaign (e.g., 7.44.7;[62] 7.80.4; 7.81.2). In medicine, the concept signifies the very opposite of *krasis*, *summetria*, and *hygieia* (health):
it is the disorder within the body caused by intrusive and destructive
external forces. In *Heracles*, the disorder that characterizes the general
situation in Thebes during the first half of the play comes to characterize the thoughts and actions of the hero himself during the second
half.

---

[61] He goes on to specify burial *nomoi* in particular.

[62] 7.44.7 is interesting for its description of a stasis-like situation, wherein members of
the same army kill one another (by mistake): ὥστε τέλος ξυμπεσόντες αὑτοῖς κατὰ πολλὰ
τοῦ στρατοπέδου, ἐπεὶ ἅπαξ ἐταράχθησαν, φίλοι τε φίλοις καὶ πολῖται πολίταις, οὐ μόνον
ἐς φόβον κατέστησαν, ἀλλὰ καὶ ἐς χεῖρας ἀλλήλοις ἐλθόντες μόλις ἀπελύοντο ('Thus in
the end, having fallen against one another throughout many parts of the camp, when
the whole army was thrown into disorder, friend against friend and citizen against
citizen, not only did they put each other into a state of fear, but they also having come
into combat with one another could scarcely be pulled apart').

Taragmos

When he first arrives on stage to discover his family in trouble, Heracles asks, ... τίν᾽ ἐς ταραγμὸν ἥκομεν; ('into what disorder have I come?' 533). And indeed, it is a disturbing scene: Heracles returns in triumph from the Underworld only to discover his family dressed in the clothing of the dead and preparing to go to the Underworld themselves, albeit by the normal route of death. The disorder of dress is only one element in a situation full of reversals: the wife outside the house, the attack of the tyrant directed against the weak (female, aged, and young) and innocent, the city in stasis, the new tyrant Lycus supported in opposition to the family of the old friend and helper Heracles. It is into this disorder that Heracles comes.

Not many lines later, however, Heracles' own plan of vengeance is described in the same terms: Amphitryon suggests to his son that he first pray to the gods and then kill Lycus with some stealth before wreaking vengeance on the citizenry at large, πόλιν δὲ σὴν / μὴ πρὶν ταράξῃς πρὶν τόδ᾽ εὖ θέσθαι, τέκνον (604–605: 'do not throw the city into disorder before you have set right this situation, son'). Thus Heracles has the ability to incite disorder (ταράξῃς) as well as to tame (ἐξημεροῦν, 20, 852). Heracles' situation is strangely similar to Lycus' at this point: the outsider[63] who, arriving in a city disrupted by violence, will use violence to establish his position. Indeed, Amphitryon has already described Lycus' pre-emptive strike against the family as a decision to 'quench murder with murder' (ὡς φόνῳ σβέσῃ φόνον, 40); now Heracles will kill Lycus in retribution not for the actual deed, but for the attempt; he will rectify this *taragmos* with *taragmos*. The difference

---

[63] Heracles' position in Thebes is an odd one: at the beginning of the play, Argos is called his *patra* (18); at the end, his *patra* is Thebes (1285). Moreover, Heracles is no Cadmeian either, but derives his claim to Theban power by virtue of his marriage to Megara and the benefits he has done for the city (defeating the Minyans, building an altar to Zeus, etc.). Helena Foley's discussion of the epinician aspects of this play reveals the tension between local and pan-Hellenic hero which is essential in cults of Heracles. Moreover, she points out that Attic cults of Heracles are never directly involved with city and politics: they are located in suburbs and demes of Attica; the close connection between Heracles and the Ephebes is as close as his cult comes to city cult. See Foley (1985) 174–188. In Thebes, the cult of Heracles is located within the city, but it takes the form of a stone (the stone that Athena throws at Heracles to stop his murderous activities). Heracles in Euripides' play is pulled away from his Theban context and brought to Athens—his Theban connections are not suppressed in the play, but the stress on Theban cults, geography and history is certainly less obvious than in other Theban plays such as the *Phoenissae* and the *Bacchae*.

between the two men's action lies not in the means, but in the target and the intentions: the tyrant Lycus aims to kill the innocent only for his own gain, whereas Heracles, always a servant to others despite his physical prowess, intends to punish the guilty on behalf of the innocent.[64]

The disorder that Heracles threatens to effect in Thebes soon takes over Heracles himself. Just as the *philoi* in Thebes refuse to help their *philoi*, undermining the whole concept of *philia*, and do so because stasis and tyranny have disrupted the proper rule of law within the city, so now Heracles turns on his own family, whom he himself calls *philtatoi* (most dear, 1147). Iris instructs the protesting Lyssa to drive Heracles mad, a madness which is to include παιδοκτόνους φρενῶν ταράγμους (835–836: 'child-slaying disorders of the mind'). The disorder will now exist within the body and mind of Heracles himself. Heracles reiterates this image later as he is coming to his senses after his bout of madness. Still ignorant of what he has actually done, he speaks not of *paidoktonoi taragmoi* but rather describes the disorder that has affected him:

ὡς ⟨δ'⟩ ἐν κλύδωνι καὶ φρενῶν ταράγματι
πέπτωκα δεινῷ καὶ πνοὰς θερμὰς πνέω
μετάρσι', οὐ βέβαια πλευμόνων ἄπο.   (1091–1093)

But it is as though I have fallen into a wave and a terrible
   disorder of my *phrên*
and I breathe hot breaths,
shallow ones, not deep breaths from my lungs.

Heracles perceives the madness as a natural disorder by which he has been affected and which still exists within his body. The specifically medical implications of *taragmos* here are reinforced by the mention of his breathing as *metarsia*, shallow, a description that has good credentials in medical treatises.[65]

---

[64] Konstan (1999) also observes similarities between the two men, especially in the fact that Heracles, in his madness, will aim to kill the innocent wife and children of his enemy, Eurystheus. He argues that Euripides creates these parallels as part of an exploration of the nature of the warrior, and the difficulty of integrating the ferocious values of the warrior into the domestic setting. Rehm (2000: 367 n. 16) adds that Lycus and Heracles would have been played by the same actor, a fact he argues would have been noticed by the audience and contributes to the parallelism Euripides establishes between the two figures.

[65] Cf. the parallels from medicine cited by Bond in his note *ad* 1093: *Morb. Mul.* 2.130, *Epid.* 3.1 (case 7); Galen *De difficultate respirationis* 3.11, 7.946.3–4 Kühn.

Yet a fifth use of this image of disorder is to be found in the play. Although the other instances of *taragmos* and its cognates apply variously to interior and exterior aspects of the hero (i.e., the city, his family, himself), lines 906–909, which have been assigned to different speakers by different scholars,[66] contain a usage more difficult to interpret:

Ἀμφιτρύων. ἢ ἤ· τί δρᾷς, ὦ Διὸς παῖ, μελάθρῳ;
τάραγμα ταρτάρειον, ὡς ἐπ' Ἐγκελάδῳ ποτέ, Παλλάς,
ἐς δόμους πέμπεις.

Amphitryon. Ah, ah: what are you doing, child of Zeus, to the house?
A hellish disaster, Pallas, as you once did against Enceladus,
you send against the house.

The *taragma tartareion* has been variously interpreted as either a stone or an earthquake used by Athena to stop Heracles' mad rampage. Her actions are compared in this passage to her treatment of Enceladus, one of the Giants whom she defeated in the Battle of the Gods and Giants. In Euripides' *Ion* 209–211, the chorus admiring the temple of Apollo at Delphi mentions the metopes that show Athena fighting Enceladus and indicate that she is brandishing a shield against him in this particular visual representation. Other traditions recount that Athena defeated Enceladus by throwing Sicily on top of him: under Mt. Aetna he still lies, powerless but occasionally breathing out fiery breaths.[67] Taken together with the account given by the messenger at lines 1002–1004,[68] it seems clear that Athena definitely arrives and stops Heracles with a stone—an object smaller than Sicily, of course, but still an action structurally similar to her action against Enceladus. Yet *taragma tartareion* is a very strange expression for a stone, that most inanimate of objects. The chorus has only just described (905) a *thyella* (storm, squall, disturbance) shaking the house, yet the comparison to Enceladus seems

---

[66] The lines have also been attributed to the chorus (by Wilamowitz). Wilamowitz later changed his mind and gave the lines to Amphitryon. See the discussion of Bond, pp. 304–305.

[67] Could there be a further similarity between Heracles and Enceladus expressed in just those very lines discussed above where the waking Heracles describes the disorder which he has suffered and describes himself as breathing out *pnoas thermas*? Moreover, he has been tied down and rendered physically powerless at this point.

[68] ἀλλ' ἦλθεν εἰκών, ὡς ὁρᾶν ἐφαίνετο
Παλλάς, κραδαίνουσ' ἔγχος †ἐπὶ λόφῳ κέαρ†
κἄρριψε πέτρον στέρνον εἰς Ἡρακλέους, ...
But an image came, Pallas as it was revealed to those who saw,
brandishing a spear, with a plumed helmet,
and she threw a rock at the chest of Heracles ...

to preclude an exact identification between the house-shaking and the *taragma*—Athena did not destroy Enceladus with an earthquake. The ambiguity of the phrase is perhaps deliberate: Amphitryon, who most probably speaks these lines, cannot in all the confusion define exactly what Athena is doing, but rather combines several events into one horrible disorder. If this interpretation is correct, then it seems possible to hear in these words yet a further implication: the *taragma tartareion* is also Heracles himself. After all, with the exception of the very first usage in the play, all the *tarag-* words have been applied to Heracles and his actions. Moreover, *tartareion* is appropriate to Heracles in that he has just returned from the Underworld. The chorus has expressed the wish for a second life which would serve to distinguish the bad from the good (655–672), yet Heracles' return from Hades to just such a second life has revealed that differentiating between bad and good can never be rendered so easy and that a second life may not be an unmitigated good. Heracles is sent against his own house as a 'hellish disorder' which destroys not only his family but also his life of glory and renown.[69]

Metabolê

The stasis in the city and the disorder from which Heracles suffers and which he also instigates contribute a sense of instability to the play. This instability is reinforced by yet another concept emphasized in the play, that of change. Change is represented early on as a source of hope, but it quickly becomes a recipe for disaster. Thus, Amphitryon, while admitting to Megara that he has no plan to save them and little hope of rescue from the threats of Lycus, nevertheless explains that he finds hope and comfort in the very principle of change: just as the winds change, so do the fortunes of human beings.

> κάμνουσι γάρ τοι καὶ βροτῶν αἱ συμφοραί,
> καὶ πνεύματ' ἀνέμων οὐκ ἀεὶ ῥώμην ἔχει,
> οἵ τ' εὐτυχοῦντες διὰ τέλους οὐκ εὐτυχεῖς·
> ἐξίσταται γὰρ πάντ' ἀπ' ἀλλήλων δίχα.
> οὗτος δ' ἀνὴρ ἄριστος ὅστις ἐλπίσιν
> πέποιθεν αἰεί· τὸ δ' ἀπορεῖν ἀνδρὸς κακοῦ.   (101–106)

---

[69] Schamun (1997) also underscores the *taragmos* theme in *Heracles*; she argues that the *taragmos* represents Heracles' own existential crisis, as he must try to reconcile his divine and mortal parentage and the conflicting demands of his role as hero and family man. She stresses the tension between disorder and clarity that is represented in the play's emphasis on *taragmos* and *diagnosis*.

For even the misfortunes of mortals grow weary,
and the breaths of the wind do not always have strength.
Those who prosper are not prosperous through to the end:
for all things separate out apart from one another.
This man is best who always trusts in hope:
for despairing is characteristic of a cowardly man.

He repeats this argument at 215–216 when he advises Lycus to refrain from excessively violent behavior, as Lycus may end up suffering violence himself should his fortune be changed by the gods. Of course, the same principle can be applied to Heracles' own success—he, too, is subject to the winds of change. Yet neither Amphitryon nor the chorus seem cognizant of this; rather they are jubilant over the changes wrought by Heracles on his return. Μεταβολὰ κακῶν ('a change from evils') sings the chorus at 735, and, a few verses later at 765–766, μεταλλαγαὶ γὰρ δακρύων, / μεταλλαγαὶ συντυχίας ... ('exchanges of tears, exchanges of fortune'). The chorus uses the image of changing tides to describe the actions of the gods on behalf of Heracles: δίκα καὶ θεῶν παλίρρους πότμος (739: 'justice and retribution flowing back from the gods'). Heracles' return and the restoration of his power are emphasized, twice with the word *palin* (again) at 736 and 743. Later in the ode, they speak of the history of Thebes as a series of exchanges, as the city passes from generation to generation under the rule of the descendants of the Spartoi:

αὔξετ᾽ εὐγαθεῖ κελάδῳ
ἐμὰν πόλιν, ἐμὰ τείχη
σπαρτῶν ἵνα γένος ἐφάνθη,
χαλκασπίδων λόχος, ὃς γᾶν
τέκνων τέκνοις μεταμείβει,
Θήβαις ἱερὸν φῶς.   (792–797)

Extol with glad song
my city, my walls
where the race of the Spartoi appeared,
a band of bronze-shielded warriors, who
continually hand over the land from children to children,
a holy light for Thebes.

These words suggest that Thebes, despite the instability stressed elsewhere in the play, has through a series of equal exchanges (Spartoi children for Spartoi children) remained unchanged throughout these generations—the differences between all these children are erased. The substitution, exchange or replacement of Lycus by Heracles is also stressed, with only two major distinctions between the two figures addressed directly: Heracles is the old lord,[70] Lycus the new, and Heracles is of better birth, stronger:

> βέβακ' ἄναξ ὁ καινός, ὁ δὲ παλαίτερος
> κρατεῖ, λιμένα λιπών γε τὸν Ἀχερόντιον.   (769–770)

The new lord has gone, the earlier one
prevails, having left behind the shores of Acheron.

> κρείσσων μοι τύραννος ἔφυς
> ἢ δυσγένει' ἀνάκτων,   (809–810)

You were born a stronger tyrant for me
than [Lycus] the illborn of lords.

These issues of change and exchange are emphasized by the action of the play, which of course depicts the altering fortunes of Heracles' family. Strohm has analyzed the course of the play in terms of a series of surprises and reversals: among the most compelling are the return of Heracles, the rescue of the family, the killing of Lycus, the onset of Heracles' madness, the arrival of Theseus and the decision by Heracles to live.[71]

A series of inversions reinforces this element of surprise and uncertainty. Megara, the woman, argues in male terms (ἐμοί τε μίμημ' ἀνδρὸς οὐκ ἀπωστέον, 294: 'I must not refuse to imitate a man') for the glory of a dignified death against the weaker hopes of the old man Amphitryon; while she argues for decisiveness and action of a sort, he resorts to philosophizing. Amphitryon himself argues with Lycus against traditional hoplite warfare and for the safer and more individual method of bow and arrow fighting.[72] The youth of Thebes, instead of supporting the very hero whom they are customarily supposed to emulate and admire in Greek society, turn against him and support the man of poor

---

[70] Although this is not true in the strictest sense, since Creon is actually the older lord. It should be noted that in line 769, καινός is a widely accepted substitution for the manuscript reading κλεινός. Basset (1996) maintains that the manuscript reading here (and at 735–733 and 745–746) should be retained, arguing that each of the original readings can be interpreted in such a way that the play consistently refers to Lycus as the old king and Heracles as the new. Basset suggests that Heracles' rule is legitimated therefore largely through merit, not heredity, making the ensuing scenes of madness all the more tragic (14).

[71] Strohm (1957) 108–110.

[72] In an extensive analysis of the significance of the bow, Michelini (1987: 242–246) shows how Amphitryon's argument fits into the larger themes of the play (with its emphasis on different brands of heroism); she also points out how Euripides stresses the bow in Heracles' speech near the end of the play (265–266).

birth, Lycus.[73] The family of Heracles dresses in the clothes of the dead before they actually die—presumably the staging reveals a sharp contrast between the virile Heracles returning from the land of the dead in his traditional costume of lion skin, bow and arrow, and club, and his family preparing to go there in death, already in the clothes of the dead. Lyssa rationally argues against Iris that it makes no sense to treat Heracles so terribly—even Madness (Lyssa) argues against madness (847–854). Heracles, who proclaims as his last words on stage that everyone loves their children (636) and urges his family to trust him (624–628), kills them without pity. At the end of the play, Heracles becomes dependent on Theseus, whom he had previously rescued; although Theseus persuades Heracles to live by giving him the opportunity to be a benefactor to the Athenians, it is clear within the action of the play itself that Heracles and Theseus have changed places in the power hierarchy—Theseus now has the position of greater power. Heracles himself admits as much at 1423–1424, using once again the image of the *epholkides* (little boats) with which he had previously described his relationship to his children (631–632). Yet all these reversals bring about no real healing: although Heracles decides to "endure life," he is hardly restored to his former self. At the end of the play, Theseus explains to Heracles that he is not now the famous Heracles since he is sick (ὁ κλεινὸς Ἡρακλῆς οὐκ εἶ νοσῶν, 1414). *Metabolê* alone is not a sufficient cure.

Prognosis

Change may indeed bring about good, it may be quite positive, but it is unpredictable. Prediction, hope and expectation all play a role in the changing fortunes of the *Heracles*. So much is beyond expectation, beyond what could have been predicted. Early in the play, Megara criticizes, and Amphitryon defends, reliance on hope rather than on plan-

---

[73] This division of young and old is not stated explicitly, but the oft-stated wish of the members of the chorus that they could be young and strong again so that they could fight for Heracles and his family implies that the young men of the city are not helping Heracles. This conflict has a contemporary historical parallel in the competition between the older Nicias and the younger Alcibiades; in Thucydides, when the two debate the Sicilian policy (6.8.4–6.23), Nicias appeals to the faction of older men against younger men, whereas Alcibiades argues against such divisiveness, appealing to the common interests of all Athenian citizens. See the discussion of de Romilly (1976), who pays special attention to the use of medical theory in the speeches.

ning and rational knowledge; they speak of Heracles' return as beyond expectation. Thus, Amphitryon speaks of 'despair of safety' (ἀπορία σωτηρίας) at 54, even though he argues at 105–106 that a good man always has hope, whereas *aporia* characterizes the bad man. Megara speaks of hopes for safety (80–81 and 84–85), although indicating that she expects there is none. When Amphitryon can only suggest delay as a remedy for their evils (87 and especially 93: ἐν ταῖς ἀναβολαῖς τῶν κακῶν ἔνεστ' ἄκη, 'in delays exist remedies for evils') and asserts he will continue to rely on hope (91), Megara criticizes his thinking: although she too would love to remain hopeful, δοκεῖν δὲ τἀδόκητ' οὐ χρή, γέρον (92: 'one must not count on the unexpected, old man'). As they prepare at last to meet their deaths, even Amphitryon loses hope: delay cannot save hope, he says at 506–507, and nothing is secure (511–512). They are both utterly amazed by the return of Heracles; Amphitryon, almost speechless (*aphasia*, 515), is unable to describe, to enunciate rationally what he sees. The triumph of Heracles, who has finally completed the labors celebrated in detail by the chorus in the second stasimon, reaches a pitch of excitement with the killing of Lycus and the rescue of the family. It is here, as we have seen, that the chorus sings so emphatically of *metabolê* and *metallagê*. Yet they also stress that the fulfillment of their hopes could not have been predicted: δοκημάτων ἐκτὸς ἦλθεν ἐλπίς (771: 'hope has come beyond expectations').

The wild swings from gloom to joy should probably awaken in the audience a sense of fear rather than confidence in the rational order of the world. For Greek attitudes towards change included the notion that tragic reversals could easily occur just when a person was at his or her most fortunate.[74] Indeed, the chorus responds to the appearance of Lyssa and Iris with the words ταχὺ τὸν εὐτυχῆ μετέβαλεν δαίμων (884: 'swiftly has the daimon changed the conditions of the fortunate man'). Heracles, in a passage whose authenticity for this play has been disputed (1291–1293),[75] states that changes are grievous for those who

---

[74] Cf. *Aphorisms* 1.3 on the particular danger of changes in health for athletes. Traditional narratives, such as the story of Solon and Croesus in Herodotus *Histories* 1.29–33 with its moral, 'call no one happy until he is dead,' (1.32.7) exemplify this belief in the potential perils of good fortune. Although Herodotus' Solon maintains that the most fortunate man is the one who dies old, having served his city well and having prospered with respect to his family, he cites the story of Cleobis and Biton as one of great good fortune: these two men died young, but in glorious circumstances.

[75] These lines are deleted by some scholars not because they are un-Euripidean, but because they contradict the basic point of the speech in which they currently stand. Heracles argues in this speech that he has never been fortunate, not even in

are fortunate; those who have never know good fortune are in some way better off. Sophisticated thinkers such as the medical writers claim that prognosis, the ability to predict the course of events through an understanding of the ways of nature and a systematic analysis of signs and symptoms, is one of the great advantages of the rationalist *logoi* they construct; yet such a capacity is conspicuously lacking in *Heracles*. The only successful prediction is based on augury: Heracles has come secretly into the city, he explains, because he saw a bird and interpreted it as an omen of some problem at home (596–598). Yet even this bird of omen does not forestall so very much—indeed, Heracles undermines the value of the omen in practically the same breath, when he asserts that he doesn't care (μέλει μὲν οὐδὲν, 595) if the whole city has seen him.[76]

As much as the characters in the play seem to cry out for the ability to prognosticate, to predict the future, diagnosis and understanding of what actually occurs is terrifying.[77] Knowledge of what he has done brings only tremendous grief to the hero: the remedy for ignorance, the cure for which he asks at 1107 (δύσγνοιαν ὅστις τὴν ἐμὴν ἰάσεται;, 'who will cure my ignorance?'), seems far worse than the disease of ignorance itself. Amphitryon tries to avoid giving Heracles knowledge of anything beyond his own body, which has been bound, a disgrace in itself (1123–1125). Yet Heracles insists that silence will not do—he wants to know (1126). Knowledge, however, brings only pain and misery, not power or happiness. Small wonder, then, that Heracles can see no other ending for himself (and thus for the play) than death: the only choice left to

---

his infancy—thus, it makes no sense for him to speak of change in fortune from good to bad or otherwise. Bond *ad* 1291–1293 that these particular lines could still remain as a general reflection on good and bad fortune; however, lines 1299–1300 must go.

[76] Scholars have criticized the introduction of the bird as the intrusion of Euripidean rationalism, pointing to his penchant for over-explaining certain dramatic conveniences and conventions (cf. Bond *ad* 595–598)—yet Euripides' purpose is perhaps rather to underscore the characters' inability to prognosticate successfully even when they claim such an ability. Even if one does not see such a moment as evidence of artistic failure, it is, surely, an example of the Euripidean detail that calls attention to the creative hand of the poet at work, rather than disguising the fact of authorship. Certainly the earlier words of Heracles at his entrance give no hint that he is arriving in secrecy.

[77] This is a familiar paradox in Greek tragedy. Those who actually can foresee the future, such as Cassandra, are certainly no happier or more successful than those who do not have this ability. Those who attempt to control the future once they have learned something about it also seem doomed to failure: witness, of course, Oedipus in the *Oedipus Tyrannus*.

him is among alternative forms of dying (1148–1152).[78] Knowledge para-doxically moves him from light to darkness, as first a 'cloud' of groans envelops him (1140), and a few verses later he covers his head so as to avoid polluting Theseus (1159–1162) and the sun (1231). The man who returned from the darkness of Hades now seeks darkness to cover him.[79]

The inversions, the surprises, the irrational events, and the focus on the human inability to prognosticate emphasize human powerlessness; scientific thinking is rendered inadequate to the demands of this tragic situation. Although all the characters in *Heracles* seek in some way to define and control the action, they are repeatedly frustrated in these attempts by other forces, human and divine, which prevent any individual from attaining his own personal desires—except, that is, for Theseus, representative of the Athenian polis, who manages to convince Heracles to renounce ideas of suicide and come to Athens.

Madness and healing

It is already clear, I hope, from my analysis of stasis, *taragmos*, *metabolê*, and the inability to prognosticate, that this play presents a ready supply of diseases and a lack of proficient healers. The delay which Amphit-ryon hopes will bring a cure fails ultimately to do so, for Heracles kills Megara and the children himself. As we have seen, Amphitryon's trust in the power of nature to heal does have good medical credentials, yet his version of this idea is somewhat problematic. Amphitryon main-tains that nature is characterized by mutability, that change is nature's constant and that such instability is a source of hope for those in trou-ble (101–106). Yet, although Amphitryon is arguing that nature has the power to cure the troubles of Heracles' family if only they wait long enough, he is not doing so on the basis of careful observation, rea-soned diagnosis, and hopeful prognosis, but out of despair; the path from identification of cause has not led to efficacious remedy and

---

[78] Strong parallels exist here between *Heracles* and Sophocles' *Aias*: both protagonists are driven mad at divine instigation and, upon awakening from the typical post-madness sleep, both are informed of their actions by sympathetic relatives, Tecmessa in *Aias* and Amphitryon here. Both contemplate suicide once they learn what they have done. However, here the contrast begins, as Theseus arrives in time to prevent Heracles from taking his own life, whereas Teucrus comes too late to do the same for Aias (although it is unclear, of course, whether he would have been able to achieve a rescue even if he had been able to speak to Aias).

[79] On aspects of visibility and invisibility in the play, see Padilla (1992).

no reasonable alternative presents itself. Moreover, when Amphitryon remarks that ἐξίσταται γὰϱ πάντ' ἀπ' ἀλλήλων δίχα (104: 'all things separate out apart from one another'), his words resonate neither with Hippocratic notions of health (with their emphasis on *krasis*) nor with standard political theories of the healthy state (characterized by *eukosmia* and *homonoia*)—indeed, his words ironically remind us of the polarized political situation in Thebes.

Amphitryon relies on the impersonal hand of nature to remedy the situation because it seems that help cannot be expected from either the gods or other human beings. No divine order and no human healer is prepared to save them. On the other hand, the troubles from which they suffer are entirely human in origin: both stasis and tyranny are a product of Theban society and Theban nature. When Heracles returns from his labors, he does not rail at the gods for failing to protect his family; rather, he is angry at the Thebans' disloyalty, their lack of gratitude for the benefits he has conferred on them (558–560). Determined to save his family from destruction and to punish both Lycus and the Thebans, he exits the stage insisting on the universality of human nature; despite some differences, everyone loves their children (633–636). And Heracles places himself squarely in that group of human beings. His reappearance from Hades may be miraculous, but it is as a domestic family man that he assumes the role of rescuer. A human rescuer to remedy the situation caused by other humans.

However, as I have discussed above, the disorder (*taragmos*) that characterizes Thebes in the first part of the play becomes centered on Heracles' own person. Immediately after the death of Lycus, Iris and Lyssa unexpectedly appear above the house and Iris directs Lyssa to drive Heracles mad. Surely there is no clearer instance of direct divine causality of disease in tragedy. As Iris announces at her arrival, she has come not to bring harm (βλάβος) against the entire city, but rather to do battle (στρατεύομεν) against only one man (824–825).[80] Such an intention runs counter to the narrative situation common in many tragic plots (including Homer), wherein the suffering of the leader or king brings suffering upon his subjects—whether the latter are guilty or innocent (e.g., the plagues in the *Iliad* and the *Oedipus Tyrannus*, which come about because of the wrongful actions of Agamemnon and Oedi-

---

[80] A rather inverted use of language here: one might expect battles to be fought against a city and harm to be brought against one man. Iris' words indicate that the political concerns of the play have turned to focus on Heracles.

pus respectively). Here, the gods explicitly intervene after the humans
have set into motion a specifically human form of destruction, stasis; this disease, unlike the madness of Heracles, has as its root cause
human social problems. At the same time, I have argued that Heracles
adds, or at the very least intends to add to the disorder in Thebes by
killing all unfriendly Theban citizens, and he states this intention before
the intervention of the gods. Heracles is then driven mad and suffers
disorders of the mind. Euripides, I believe, does not mean us to think
that Heracles is mad before the arrival of the goddesses, as Wilamowitz
argued; rather, Heracles' actions towards the Thebans are deliberately
separated from his actions towards his family, and his decision to kill
the Thebans is made while he is thinking rationally. Whether he actually carries out his stated intentions is left very unclear. Only later and
very briefly (966–967) do the words of Amphitryon suggest to the audience that perhaps Heracles has killed others besides Lycus: Amphitryon
asks, οὔ τί που φόνος σ᾽ ἐβάκχευσεν νεκρῶν / οὓς ἄρτι καίνεις; ('surely the
killing of the corpses whom you have just now killed has not somehow
driven you mad?')—the plural (νεκρῶν οὕς) indicates that more than
the single death of Lycus is meant here.[81] However, the audience knows
who and what is responsible for the madness of Heracles: according to
the action of the play, the gods are, but perhaps we are meant to ask
ourselves nonetheless about the rationality behind political discord.

There are other implications in Iris' argument that she and Lyssa
have come to do battle not against the city, but against only one man.
For in the case of Heracles, such a division between the well-being of
the individual and the well-being of his community is problematic. As
even Lyssa points out, Heracles is conspicuous for his good deeds; he
has served the interests of both humans and gods (849–853). Indeed,
Thebes will lose this *euergetês* (as Heracles is called at 877, 1252, and
1309) because of his divinely-induced madness. Both madness and pollution are isolating, although for very different reasons. Madness cuts
the sufferer off from his surroundings because he does not perceive

---

[81] Bond (p. 315) comments on this passage that Amphitryon's 'suggestion is a weak
one, for Heracles has killed many villains in his time … One may quote against
it *Ion* 1334 καθαρὸς ἅπας τοι πολεμίους ὃς ἂν κτάνῃ ["everyone is pure who kills
their enemies," *my translation*].' While Bond may be right about the weakness of the
suggestion, surely the statement from *Ion* is not to be taken as the only Greek attitude
towards killing enemies—indeed, plays like *Troades* or *Orestes* urge us to consider possible
contexts in which such action is not justified. Furthermore, the issue of killing one's
fellow citizens is surely rather different than killing someone from another city.

the same world as those around him; the madman lives in a world of his own making. Those who watch Heracles go mad wonder at first whether he is playing a game (952); yet they have no fear that they themselves will become mad, too. Thus, Amphitryon actually touches Heracles as he tries to determine what is affecting his son's mind (963–964). Pollution, however, isolates because it is contagious: until the polluted individual is purified, his or her presence is a direct and communicable threat to the society. In his dialogue with Theseus, Heracles imagines a life of isolation in Thebes, prevented from participation in communal life because of his polluted state (1281–1284). His own experience now tells him that not even the best and strongest of individuals is immune to madness, and that all human beings are capable of wreaking havoc upon one another.

Theseus' response to Heracles' assessment of his situation is at once very practical and quite radical. He attributes the madness of Heracles to divine intervention while denying the actuality of pollution. He rejects the contagious aspect of pollution entirely: friends cannot pollute their friends (1234), and those same gods whose immoral exploits he recounts (1315–1319) are impervious to human pollution (1232). He offers very little by way of consolation, suggesting only that since the gods themselves do bad things (according to the stories of poets, which may or may not be true),[82] Heracles should not worry so much about his own misfortune, but bear up and go on with his life (1314–1321). Indeed, he implies with the word *hyperpheu* (too much, 1321) that Heracles' grief-stricken reaction is excessive. Admittedly, there is perhaps very little one can say to console a person in Heracles' situation; nevertheless, the examples Theseus gives of divine misbehavior are hardly comparable in magnitude to what Heracles has done. While he acknowledges the enormity of Heracles' crimes, he sees no need for Heracles to be isolated from the human community. Indeed, Theseus not only speaks with and touches his friend, but he wishes to bring him to Athens where a cult will be established for him after his death (1331–1335). He is able to convince Heracles that living is an option and is in fact the choice of a brave man, because he can still be useful to society, specifically Athenian society. If Heracles comes to Athens, says Theseus, he will be given gifts. Even greater honors will come after his death, when Athenians will make dedications and sacrifices to him

---

[82] Bond points out that the use of εἴπερ in 1315 means that Theseus thinks these stories are true.

(1331–1333). The Athenians will benefit as well, gaining a beautiful victory crown in exchange for accepting and helping the outcast Heracles (1334–1335).

Theseus is not blasphemous, but he sees the need for a united human front in the face of capricious divine activity. Theseus' interpretation of the situation correlates with the 'miasmatic' conception of disease discussed earlier:[83] because madness is attributed to the gods, the human response can be one of sympathy; moreover, the human community can unite in order to find a solution to the suffering caused by these irrational forces of pain.[84] When disease attacks the good or the innocent, society must act not to isolate them but to restore them to health and to reintegrate them into the healthy community. Theseus urges Heracles to leave Thebes 'for the sake of custom' (τοῦ νόμου χάριν, 1322) and come to Athens where he will be purified—human custom requires purification. But Theseus' insistence on contact with the polluted man shows that he does not consider pollution to exist materially. Moreover, the madness and the crimes committed under the influence of madness do not erase the beneficial acts that Heracles has done for humankind: after death, he will be worthy of a cult because of his good reputation and his fame, his *eukleia*.

Theseus appears to provide the most effective treatment that this play will admit: he succeeds in convincing Heracles to live, but he hardly restores him to health. In the final set of stichomythia in the play, Theseus' participation in the doctor model I have discussed earlier is most fully revealed. Here, he exhibits a blend of sympathy and authority: he helps Heracles, now weak in limb (1395) and broken in spirit, to his feet and encourages him to accept his support; at the same time, he ignores or rejects the expressed wishes of his patient. Thus, at 1397–1398, when Heracles seems ready to renew his expressions of grief, Theseus says simply, παῦσαι ('stop'), and offers him physical support. At 1406–1407, when Heracles asks to look at his children one more time, Theseus replies: ὡς δὴ τί; φίλτρον τοῦτ' ἔχων ὁράων ἔσῃ; ('for what purpose then? having this as a remedy will you ease your pain?'). The phrase *raiôn einai* occurs in the Hippocratic Corpus to express treatment which eases pain but does not actually cure the disease,[85]

---

[83] See p. 105 note 9.
[84] On the power of human friendship as the one positive 'message' of the play, see Gregory (1992) 121–154.
[85] See Van Brock (1961) 212–213.

and the concept of *philtron*, as mentioned in Part I, has no place in sophisticated medicine; thus, Theseus' words are those of a rationalist, dismissing the misguided notions of his patient. When Heracles protests against Theseus' dismissive attitude, Theseus reminds him at 1414 that, being sick, he is no longer the renowned Heracles he was at the start of the drama.

The play does not completely vindicate the views of either Heracles or Theseus with respect to the nature of the gods, pollution, disease and healing. Although Heracles' madness may be caused (at least most obviously) by divinities and his pollution remedied by human social institutions, the other disease of this play, stasis, has its causes only in the nature of human beings. Indeed the play reveals Theseus' view of human nature as rather optimistic.[86] That very society on which Theseus relies to close ranks against the irrational forces of madness and disease is subject to the disease of civic strife: sick, divided by factionalism, weakened by greed. And we never learn how this disease is to be cured. The chaotic political situation in Thebes, so carefully outlined in the beginning of the play, suddenly disappears when Lycus is murdered. The tensions between old and young, rich and poor, which have contributed to the disease of stasis in the city, simply vanish from the discourse. Instead, the play focuses entirely on the personal suffering of Heracles and the role of Athens in healing him. Thebes' only role at the end of the play is to mourn.[87]

Stasis is always a negative phenomenon in our literary sources, aptly called a disease because of its corrosive power. If explicit discussion of stasis vanishes from *Heracles*, this does not mean that Thebes has found peace; rather, the play itself participates in the great changes and reversals that the characters suffer, and it changes its focus, proceeding not smoothly but through a series of surprises and disruptions. The play begins with a broad canvas, portraying the suffering of Thebes and of Heracles' family, but then focuses in to consider the sufferings of only one man. If divine forces are instrumental in causing Heracles' madness and suffering, human social institutions are in some way able

---

[86] On this brand of rationalism in Euripides, see Mastronarde (1986).

[87] This situation may provide a slight corrective to Griffith's contention that choruses and minor characters always survive the disasters of tragedy (1995: 119–124). While the play certainly proves his argument about the valorization of elite institutions such as *xenia*, it seems to do so at some cost: Heracles has neither protected his own family nor has he unequivocally rescued Thebes.

to help him to live, if not to live happily.[88] The question that remains unanswered is how human social institutions can cure problems of their own making. In *Heracles*, stasis is cured by a trick of language and of dramaturgy: it is simply silenced. But the historical reality of stasis in the fifth century was not so easily dispensed with.

c. Phoenissae: *Balanced interiors*

The *Phoenissae* confronts us with scenes of intra-familial conflict; it explores configurations of the human *physis* and the extent to which the qualities of an individual are universal, inherited or particular. An essential problem for the family of Oedipus is that its members are far too like each other. Jocasta and Oedipus are at once husband and wife, mother and son, and their children, products of incest, are Oedipus' brothers and sons, daughters and sisters. Too many identities and kin-ships are crowded into each single human form—and yet, the sons of Oedipus seem to insist on further crowding.[89] Eteocles and Polyneices vie to be in the same place, to hold the same position, each insisting on the different nature of the other and yet claiming the same identity as legitimate ruler of Thebes. By contrast, the sons of Creon, Haemon and Menoeceus, remain distinct: Menoeceus recognizes how he differs from his brother and thus sacrifices himself willingly for the good of the city, dying so that the city and his family may live. Tiresias states

---

[88] Sourvinou-Inwood (2003: 375–376) argues that the ancient audience will not have seen Heracles as a 'wholly innocent victim of divine malice' because of the very nature of Heracles, the hero of excess who crossed and confounded so many boundaries. Furthermore, the audience's knowledge of Heracles' later deification will help them realize that the divine order, unknowable to humans, will 'compensate' for Heracles' suffering in the present: the audience will thus be able to place Heracles' suffering in a wider perspective. This may be true, but it is not part of the discourse of the play itself. She also rightly stresses that the explanation for the madness in the play is 'complex and shifting.'

[89] On this theme of doubled and mingled identities, see Zeitlin (1990) esp. 134–139. My interpretation of *Phoenissae* as a play that focuses on identity and difference has been stimulated by Zeitlin's article and by Foley (1985). Foley's work is in turn explicitly formulated as a response to the work of Girard (1972) on sacrifice. Girard argues that sacrifice functions to preserve and/or to restore identities threatened by loss of clarity and difference (e.g., the difference between animals and humans). I would only point out that political and civil equality should not be seen as an evil in need of remedy through hierarchy or enforced difference. Rather, excessive loss or lack of separate identities, as occurs in Thebes, can result in chaos and tragedy.

that the family of Creon is 'unmixed' or 'pure' (ἀκέραιος, 943), meaning that they stem directly from the Spartoi and have not intermar-
ried with other clans or families. Menoeceus meets the qualifications
for an acceptable sacrifice because of the purity of his family and his
own unmarried, unbetrothed status. The stated purity of Creon and his
family contrasts of course with the excessive intermingling of the Labdacids. Yet even in the case of Menoeceus, there is a hint of something
troubling: the young man states that he was nursed by his aunt Jocasta
because his mother died when he was still an infant (987–988). This
detail of Menoeceus' youth is apparently unique to Euripides' account,
prompting us to ask why it is included.[90] Although it was not uncommon for a baby to be suckled by a woman other than his mother,
the task was often given to nurses unrelated to the child's family (and
indeed we have many nurses cropping up in Greek literature, such as
Eurycleia in the *Odyssey* and Cilissa in *Choephoroi*). Jocasta's role as wet
nurse to her nephew contributes to the overall sense of excessive close-
ness within the ruling family of Thebes. Thus even the pure Menoeceus
has been implicated in the impurity of the ruling family.

Menoeceus makes this statement in the intimate setting of a conversation with his father, a conversation in which the ties of immediate
family are privileged over the claims of the state (963–967). The son
assures the father that he will flee Thebes and so save himself (977–
989). However, when Creon leaves the stage believing in his son's assur-
ances, Menoeceus announces his readiness to die. He will not betray
the country which gave him birth: τοὐμὸν δ' οὐχὶ συγγνώμην ἔχει / προ-
δότην γενέσθαι πατρίδος ἤ μ' ἐγείνατο (995–996: 'but in my case this is
not forgivable, to become a traitor to the country which gave me birth').
Menoeceus thus separates himself publicly from the private interests—
and moreover the birth claims—of his family; in order to divorce himself from the families of Creon and Jocasta, he claims the land itself
as his progenitor. But Menoeceus cannot escape participation in the
tragic destruction of his own family, inasmuch as his self-imposed separation means in this case his death. Moreover, although he apparently

---

[90] Menoeceus does need an excuse to delay his departure as he hides his true
intentions from his father. But surely there were many other plausible excuses available
to the playwright. The story of Jocasta's nursing is certainly unusual enough to evoke
some curiosity in the audience. Mastronarde *ad loc.* and *ad* 965 links the story to the
theme of kinship so prominent in the play and argues that it contributes to the contrast
between the attitudes of Jocasta and Creon towards each other's children.

saves the city from utter destruction through his act of self-sacrifice,[91] he fails to preserve the ruling family and the aunt who nursed him as a baby.

The circumstances surrounding the sacrifice of Menoeceus participate in the issues of identity and difference raised by the play in still another way. In explaining that the earth demands the sacrifice as recompense for the loss of Ares' dragon slain by Cadmus many years before, Tiresias describes the process as an exchange of equals: fruit for fruit, blood for blood (χθὼν δ' ἀντὶ καρποῦ καρπὸν ἀντί θ' αἵματος / αἷμ' ἢν λάβῃ βρότειον, 937–938: 'if the land takes fruit for fruit and mortal blood in exchange for blood'). Yet the benefits of such an act are set forth in a play where the exchange of equals yields only conflict and destruction, whether in the seven battles at the seven gates, where Argive and Theban heroes are perfectly matched against one another, or again in the denser knot of exchanges and equalities exemplified by the family of Oedipus itself. The issue of total equality is central to the play; indeed it is the *Phoenissae* in which Jocasta essays a discourse on the merits of *Isotês* (equality).[92]

In Jocasta's discussion of this theme (528–585, esp. 535–554), she praises sharing, equality and moderate behavior, and she asserts the value of *Isotês* by resorting to examples of equal rule in the natural world (e.g., sun and moon). Her argument surely seems eminently reasonable to a modern audience, particularly one whose members are committed to a democratic system. The ancient audience of *Phoenissae*, produced most likely in 410 or 409,[93] had in 411 experienced the

---

[91] Menoeceus' noble self-sacrifice does not receive much notice in the rest of the play (particularly striking when we contrast the *Phoenissae* to situations of human sacrifice in *Hecabe*, *Iphigenia in Aulis*, and *Heraclidae*). However, the city of Thebes is not sacked or overrun by the attacking Argives, so it seems that his action has been to this extent effective. Yet the fate of the city, which is subject to some consideration at the start of the play in the parados and in the agon (tyranny vs. the good of the city), is largely ignored by the end of the play—it is the fate of its rulers that receives greater attention. On the function of Menoeceus' sacrifice, see Foley (1985) 132–139, 145–146; see also the perceptive analysis of Nancy (1983), stressing the pathos of human sacrifice in Euripides and noting that young innocents are called upon to die in situations of civil strife, that is, situations that mark the failure of adults to address their differences successfully. She argues that Menoeceus' willing self-sacrifice, tragic in its isolation, does serve to save the city, but I think it remains unclear what exactly is being saved.

[92] Both Diggle and Mastronarde capitalize *Isotês* in Jocasta's speech because (presumably) of its function as a personified force of nature—hence, my capitalization here.

[93] See discussion in Mastronarde's edition of *Phoenissae*, pp. 11–14.

oligarchic takeover of the Four Hundred and the ensuing rule of the Five Thousand. Many members of that audience would have been at least somewhat familiar with contemporary arguments about the merits and defects of their democratic system. The issue of equality was of utmost importance to the Athenian audience, and yet the implications of equality had never been more problematic than during the upheavals of the Peloponnesian War. Although we may be inclined to read *isotês* (whether personified or not) as something of obvious positive value, particularly when advocated by the sympathetic figure of Jocasta in this play, we should remember that the Athenians themselves were struggling with the issues of merit (or at least efficiency) versus equality. Although the wider social implications of claims for *isotês* explored in *Phoenissae* are important, I wish to focus my discussion on the issue of microcosmic, familial and even corporeal *isotês*.

Let us review some of the moments in the play which lead up to the specific introduction of the *isotês* theme. The sons of Oedipus and Jocasta had earlier decided to take turns ruling in Thebes, each holding the throne for a year at a time. Yet now Eteocles, refusing to abide by his promise, will not relinquish the throne to Polyneices; thus, Polyneices has come to take over power by force of arms. The play begins with the premise that Jocasta has decided to bring her two sons together in hopes of effecting a reconciliation. In the prologue, she prays that Zeus grant *symbasis* (coming together, agreement) to her sons (85). As she and Polyneices prepare to begin the meeting with Eteocles, Polyneices looks to her to provide a *dialysis* (breaking up, dissolution) of evils (435).[94] I would suggest that Jocasta, in acting to restore balance and equilibrium to her troubled family, is trying to be a 'doctor' here; the common use of these words for reconciliation and dissolution in medical texts point us towards this interpretation. Yet, like many of the characters discussed in Part I who act in similar capacity, Jocasta is unsuccessful in her attempts at healing. Both Polyneices and the chorus urge Jocasta to reconcile her children through a process of 'dissolving' or 'breaking apart'—they use the word διαλλάσσω (and the noun διαλλαγή) several times (436, 443, 445), which literally means

---

[94] The substantive *dialysis* appears rarely in the Hippocratic Corpus, but the verb *dialyô* is quite common: e.g., *Morb. Sacr.* 13.13; *Aer.* 7.63, 10.38; *Flat.* 8.17; *Reg.* 1.27.25; *Reg.* 2.60.4, 66.37; *Aph.* 3.17.7. Mastronarde *ad* 435 stresses the legalistic use of the word and its cognates as he reviews the uses in tragedy and other fifth-century literatures.

to 'separate out' and thus to 'solve' and to 'reconcile.'[95] Thus the process by which the fraternal quarrel is to be settled involves at once *symbasis* and *dialysis*, coming together and breaking apart. This linguistic paradox prefigures the immovable conflict of Eteocles and Polyneices: they find it impossible to do both, or even either. Moreover, as Jocasta sets the stage for the agon, urging her sons to be calm and look at one another, she seems to suggest yet another impossibility, that two *philoi* should 'come together into one' (εἰς ἓν συνελθών, 462). To be sure, she speaks metaphorically, but her words reflect a central problem of the *Phoenissae*: two people cannot occupy the same space at the same time.

In the agon proper, Polyneices, speaking first, argues for the unified, monolithic nature of truth as against the complexity of injustice. The unjust *logos* is sick—thus, out of balance, unharmonious, not properly mixed—and needs strong drugs:

> ἁπλοῦς ὁ μῦθος τῆς ἀληθείας ἔφυ,
> κοὐ ποικίλων δεῖ τἄνδιχ᾽ ἑρμηνευμάτων·
> ἔχει γὰρ αὐτὰ καιρόν· ὁ δ᾽ ἄδικος λόγος
> νοσῶν ἐν αὑτῷ φαρμάκων δεῖται σοφῶν. (469–472)

The story of truth is naturally unified and simple,
nor do just causes have need of elaborate discussions:
for they have by themselves their due measure; but the unjust case
being sick in and of itself needs complicated remedies.

No divisions or differentiations (*poikiloi*) are allowed in the unified (*haplous*) *logos* of truth. Yet Polyneices believes in the possibility of a divisible kingship and a shared kingdom—not shared at the same time (as in the Spartan tradition of two kings ruling simultaneously), but successively. He asks not for the whole, but for a part (*meros*, 486), although what he wants is the whole for part of the time. Eteocles, in reply, dismisses the existence of any form of commonality or equality, except in the words themselves:

> εἰ πᾶσι ταὐτὸ καλὸν ἔφυ σοφόν θ᾽ ἅμα,
> οὐκ ἦν ἂν ἀμφίλεκτος ἀνθρώποις ἔρις·
> νῦν δ᾽ οὔθ᾽ ὅμοιον οὔτ᾽ ἴσον βροτοῖς
> πλὴν ὀνομάσαι· τὸ δ᾽ ἔργον οὐκ ἔστιν τόδε. (499–502)

---

[95] The medical usage of διαλλάσσω in the fifth century should be noted: cf., e.g, *Morb. Sacr.* 13.19; *Aer.* 12.3, 24.3, 13.10, 23.9; *Reg.* 1.6.29; *Nat. Hom.* 5.2; *Loc. Hom.* 42.7; also διαλλαγή: *Aer.* 24.29; and διάλλαξις: *Reg.* 1.10.24.

> If the same thing was by nature beautiful and wise to
>   everyone at the same time,
> there would not be spoken quarrels among men:
> but as it is there is nothing similar or equal for mortals
> except the names: the reality is not that [i.e., similar or equal].

The possibility of a shared understanding of equality (and thus, incidentally, democracy) is inconceivable to him.[96] Anything other than sole possession of the place of power results in slavery and unmanliness (*anandria*, 509). Thus, he too argues for a kind of unity, the complete concentration of power in the hands of one person; should he surrender this power, he loses his identity, he becomes not a man.

In her speech, Jocasta attempts to set Eteocles on the path of a more righteous Greek morality. It is better to honor *Isotês*, she argues, with its binding force:

> κεῖνο κάλλιον, τέκνον,
> Ἰσότητα τιμᾶν, ἣ φίλους ἀεὶ φίλοις
> πόλεις τε πόλεσι συμμάχους τε συμμάχοις
> συνδεῖ· τὸ γὰρ ἴσον νόμιμον ἀνθρώποις ἔφυ ...   (535–538)

> That would be better, son,
> to honor *Isotês*, which always binds together friends with friends
> and cities with cities and allies with allies:
> for equality is by nature lawful for humankind ...

Syndei suggests unity, harmonious connections and at the same time a certain amount of constraint and compulsion. Jocasta in fact goes on to show not how *isotês* binds things together, but how it divides them up, assigning measures and weights and distinguishing numbers (541–542). *Isotês* is a principle of nature, which governs the calm, eternal cycle of the moon and sun (543–545). This comparison, however, avoids the very problematic nature of her two sons: they are too similar, too undifferentiated, to have such easily distinguishable identities as the sun and moon.

Jocasta next speaks against a positive evaluation of excess (τὸ πλέον, 553) as she opposes the excessive power of one man (the tyrant) against the greater value of the needs of the body politic (560–568). She then continues with a criticism of Polyneices' position (569–583). Polyneices is surely a more sympathetic character in this play than the selfish Eteocles, but he, too, wants to have more than is necessary. After all, for all his talk of exile and poverty, he has managed to establish a position

---

[96] For the interpretation of lines 501–502, I follow Mastronarde *ad loc.*

for himself in Argos through his marriage with the king Adrastos' daughter. By seeking power in Thebes, he risks losing not only Thebes but also the position he has gained in Argos (and he is risking Argive lives to do so); thus, he is pursuing a very dangerous course, rather than trying to maintain a life of equilibrium and unity.

Jocasta ends her speech with an appeal to her sons to give up excess (τὸ λίαν, 584). Her final gnome, ἀμαθία δυοῖν, / εἰς ταῦθ' ὅταν μόλητον, ἔχθιστον κακόν (584–585: 'the ignorance of two people, when they come together into the same place, is a most destructive evil'), reiterates the idea of 'coming together in the same place,' yet whereas the meeting of the two brothers was to be productive, ignorance meeting ignorance is destructive. Again, a paradox arises, in that two sames coming together result not in harmony but in conflict.

The difficulties and paradoxes traced in this review of the central agon recur elsewhere in the play. So, for example, Eteocles, ironically now promoting a principle of balance, decides on a battle strategy of setting equal against equal:

> ἔσται τάδ'· ἐλθὼν ἑπτάπυργον ἐς στόμα
> τάξω λοχαγοὺς πρὸς πύλαισιν, ὡς λέγεις,
> ἴσους ἴσοισι πολεμίοισιν ἀντιθείς.   (748–750)

> This is how it will be: having gone to the seven-gated entrance
> I will arrange the companies at the gates, as you say,
> setting equals up against equal enemies.

Yet if equal fights equal, how can either side be expected to win? One side must be stronger in order to prevail, but Eteocles' stratagem would seem to ensure either stalemate or mutual destruction. The Presocratic Heraclitus had maintained that the tension between opposites created a unified world; likewise, he argued that *harmonia* resulted from the tension of sames opposing each other, as in the case of the stringed bow or the stringed lyre (DK22 B51). The opposition of equals in *Phoenissae*, however, is not productive of harmony (whose namesake Harmonia had been forced to abandon Thebes in the mythical story of a previous Theban generation); the equal forces of the play do not wish to alternate or to maintain separate positions; they do not differentiate, but instead clash and meld into an unhealthy, destructive mixture.

Even smaller details occasionally point to this difficulty. The opposition of the boar and the lion, Tydeus and Polyneices, results in the productive act of marriage, even though the marriage between Polyneices and Adrastus' daughter ultimately involves the Argives in war (the history of the relationship between Polyneices and the Argives is explained at 410–429). Yet the clash between the brothers Eteocles and Polyneices has a more immediately tragic outcome, as we know. Thus, it is interesting to note that in the final battle they are at one point described by the messenger as two boars fighting one another (1380–1381) and, in Antigone's account, as two lions (1573). The vain and terrible battle between the two brothers, between the two sames, is thus differentiated from the fight between Polyneices and Tydeus, lion and boar, a fight of which the decisive outcome is prevented by the intervention of Adrastus. The identities of the brothers are not distinctive enough and at the same time they have identities in excess. Jocasta seeks to set them in balance, she seeks to limit their excessive behavior, but she cannot resolve the paradoxes of their natures. The curse of Oedipus, the history of strife so deeply engrained among the Thebans and the problematic nature of the brothers themselves engender the tragic conflict played out in the *Phoenissae*.

Thus far, I have focused my analysis largely on the eristic nature of the brothers Polyneices and Eteocles, a nature that reflects the city in which they were born. Thebes is a place of perpetual strife among sames, where the descendants of the Earth-born continue to fight among themselves down through the generations. Even when outsiders are introduced, such as Heracles and Lycus in *Heracles* or Adrastus and the other allies of Polyneices in *Phoenissae*, they are sucked into this vortex of internal strife; they cannot solve the quarrels in Thebes, yet neither can they escape them unscathed. Outsiders, no matter what their own nature, end up suffering death and destruction along with the Thebans. Only someone like Theseus, who removes affected individuals from the city, manages to survive encounters with Thebes.

Despite this disastrous history, the Thebans endure, trying with each new generation to avoid bloodshed, and failing utterly. As with other tragedies taking place in Thebes, so too in *Phoenissae* does Euripides employ images and concepts common in medical literature as part of his dramatic arsenal. In *Phoenissae*, as I have already suggested, Jocasta plays the role of healer as she tries to save both her sons from destruction, but she fails to find the appropriate cure. For the cause of the disease is locked away, hidden deep within the house: old, blind, angry Oedipus. It is Eteocles and Polyneices who have put him there, and he has cursed them for it. Thus they are in part responsible for their own destruction. That balance which Jocasta attempts to restore among her children is impossible to achieve with the source of disease

still within the house. Only at the end of the play, after the death of
the brothers and Jocasta, does Oedipus emerge; only at the end of the
play is he expelled from the land in a final attempt at healing. This play
uses the medical ideas of *dialysis, pharmakon, apostasis*, and homeopathy
as it traces the futile attempts of the various members of the house to
remedy the congenital disease of mutual destruction that infects them.

Oedipus' presence in the house is stressed and described in omi-
nous terms from the start of the play. As Jocasta recounts the family
history in the prologue, she provides the rather shocking information
that Oedipus has not left Thebes. She explains that, having discovered
the truth of his patricide and incestuous marriage, Oedipus has blinded
himself. However, his grown sons have locked him away, hoping that
his fortune will be forgotten—a difficult task. Oedipus, 'sick from his
fortune' (πρὸς δὲ τῆς τύχης νοσῶν, 66) has cursed his sons to 'divide the
house by a deadly sword' (68). According to the time-sharing arrange-
ment made by the brothers in response to the curse, Polyneices left
the city and Eteocles took over the throne. Yet now Eteocles refuses
to surrender power, although his year is over, and, as the play begins,
Polyneices is leading a bunch of foreigners, an Argive force, against
Thebes. Jocasta has taken it upon herself to try to reconcile the brothers, to 'loosen the quarrel' (ἔριν λύουσα, 81).

The physical entity of Thebes itself is stressed in these early stages of
the play. The 'teichoskopia' (view-from-the-walls) that follows the prologue not only stresses the brilliance of the world outside the walls—the
glint of armor, the wide, open plains[97]—but also the walls themselves.[98]
The servant assures Antigone that 'the city holds the things within
securely' (τά γ' ἔνδον ἀσφαλῶς ἔχει πόλις, 117). Yet the pictographic
orderliness[99] of the army and its leaders belies the terrible disturbance
that it represents. At the end of the scene, the servant sends Antigone
back inside the house, noting that crowds are gathering 'since confusion has entered the city' (ὡς ταραγμὸς εἰσῆλθεν πόλιν, 196). The use of

---

[97] The plains around the city are mentioned at 101 and 111; the whole passage is rich
in imagery of light and brilliance, e.g., 111, 130, 166–168, 175–176, 183.

[98] For the walls, see 114–116; 180–181. The chorus also stresses the walls as they
describe in the parados the army outside the city: 239; 245.

[99] Antigone speaks as though she were viewing a mural: thus, note especially 129–
130, ⟨ὥσπερ⟩ ἐν / γραφαῖσιν ('as in pictures') and 161–162, ὁρῶ δέ πως / μορφῆς τύ-
πωμα στέρνα τ' ἐξῃκασμένα ('I see somehow the outline of his form and the likeness of
his chest'). On the significance of the references to art in this play, see Zeitlin (1994)
171–196, who stresses the connection between these images and the theme of blind-
ness/vision in the play.

the word *taragmos* is hardly suggestive of safety and security; rather, it seems that the city has been seriously disturbed even though the besieging army has not even begun their attack. The crowd approaching the palace is in fact the chorus of Phoenician women, another group of foreigners.[100] Although barbarian, they are nonetheless able to explain their close ancestral relationship to the Theban people. Thus far, then, the walls are protecting their own people.

After the parados, Polyneices too enters the walls—and once again, Euripides emphasizes this physical barrier (261–262). Yet Polyneices' status is not so clear: although his ancestral links to Thebes are not in doubt, he has come leading a foreign army against the city; moreover, he enters the city armed and watchful, ready to attack. Reassured by the presence of altars and people, he sheathes his sword and prepares to greet his mother. Later in the scene, he indicates that the walls are for him a source of danger: only his trust in Jocasta and the agreements she has set up have induced him to enter the *teichê patrôia* (homeland walls, 366). Despite all the emphasis on walls, Thebes appears to be in fact quite permeable. Indeed, as we hear several times, it has seven gates. Yet the issue of the walls serves to heighten the play's emphasis on the people these walls encircle.[101] Internal discord is surely just as responsible for the threat to Theban existence as the external pressure of an army: the history of the city, as recounted in the choral odes, and the sacrifice demanded of Menoeceus to save the city reinforce the notion that the Thebans alone are responsible for the predicament in which they find themselves.

I have discussed earlier the arguments with which Jocasta attempts to reconcile her sons: she endeavors to bring her sons together into one, urging them to honor *isotês*, and to avoid excess. She tries to establish both a *symbasis* and a *dialysis/diallagê*, a coming-together and a breaking-apart. Her attempts at healing the breach between Polyneices and Eteocles have parallels in medicine, where healers aim to restore the balance of the body after separating out and expelling the *materia*

---

[100] Note that both the army outside the walls and the chorus of women entering are described as an *ochlos* ('host,' 'crowd'—the army at 149 and 1276, the chorus at 196).

[101] The idea that a city is essentially its people and not its walls is found in contemporary sources such as Thucydides. So Nicias at Thucydides 7.77.7: ἄνδρες γὰρ πόλις καὶ οὐ τείχη οὐδὲ νῆες ἀνδρῶν κεναί ('for men are the city and not walls nor ships empty of men'). For more on this theme, see Longo (1975). On connections made by Greek writers between walls, cities, and disease, see Kosak (2000).

peccans. Moreover, she is using gentle methods against a violent disease, a course approved by most healers in most instances. But Jocasta's efforts seem bound to fail for several reasons. First of all, there is the difficulty of attempting to bring together and to break apart at the same time. Jocasta is defeated by the nature of language (which, as Polyneices points out at 471–472, is itself 'sick,' at least in its unjust form).[102] Secondly, of course, there is the nature of the brothers themselves: to some extent, they *are* the *materia peccans*, because they are excessive in their very beings. Furthermore, the brothers are not particularly good patients;[103] while professing an interest in the solutions that their mother tries to provide, they both remain fixed in their own positions. Eteocles and Polyneices have already made the mistake of locking up their father; now, they continue to make poor choices, choosing harsh methods as against the gentler ones recommended by their mother. As Eteocles points out, Polyneices too is trying to achieve a *diallagê*— but by force of arms (χϱῆν δ' αὐτὸν οὐχ ὅπλοισι τὰς διαλλαγάς, / μῆτεϱ, ποιεῖσθαι, 515–516: 'he should not make reconcilations with weapons, mother'). Thirdly, Jocasta seems destined to fail because she focuses her efforts on the sons, while overlooking the significance of their father's presence in the city. Her own language betrays the danger that he represents: twice she describes him as sick, angry and destructive (66–67; 327–336). Yet we do not meet Oedipus until after the death of Jocasta and the brothers; only at the end of the play is he expelled from the land in a kind of healing *apostasis*.

During most of the play, Oedipus remains 'hidden in darkness' (336), a source of danger that can neither see nor be seen. The actions of the brothers become the symptoms of his presence, as they inevitably carry out the terms of his curse. The characters reiterate the fate of Oedipus

---

[102] On the problematic nature of language in the play, see Soter (1993) ch. 3, esp. 97–127; 142–144. Mastronarde *ad loc*. points out that, although disease metaphors are common in tragedy, this is the only extant passage where *logos* itself is 'sick.'

[103] The author of the treatise *The Art* argues that when medicine fails to operate successfully, the fault more likely lies with the patient who has failed to follow the healer's prescriptions, rather than the healer, who after all knows what he is doing. Patients, he explains, are impatient; sick and frustrated by their disease, they do things they shouldn't do—they try to heal themselves even though they are ignorant of the proper methods of healing (7.2–5). Jouanna (commentary *ad* 7.2) notes that the disobedience of the sick is a common preoccupation among Hippocratic authors and cites *Prorrhetics* 2.4, where the author provides some methods for detecting patient noncompliance.

throughout the play, contrasting his clever handling of the Sphinx and his former fame to his current blindness and invisibility. Thus, at 763–765, Eteocles disparages his father for *amathia* (ignorance), now that Oedipus is blind, and expresses his anger over his father's curse; Eteocles then designates Creon as the executor of his wishes should he die in the approaching combat—Oedipus is apparently incapable of doing so. The choral ode that ensues gives a concise version of Oedipus' history, mentioning his expulsion at childhood, conspicuous because of the pins in his feet (804–805), then the destructive actions of the Sphinx (806–811), and finally the unlawful children produced by a polluted, incestuous marriage (815–817, admittedly, corrupt lines, but their import is clear). Tiresias, too, takes up the theme, although he is less concerned with the entire history of the city than the chorus is.[104] Tiresias maintains that the true threat to Thebes is not the besieging Argive army, but rather the sickness innate to the land, the origin of which is the family of the Labdacids. He states that the land has long been sick (νοσεῖ γὰρ ἥδε γῆ πάλαι, 867) since the time when Laius fathered Oedipus against the will of the gods. Oedipus' blindness, according to Tiresias, was supposed to be an 'example to Greece' (871). But Eteocles and Polyneices completely misread the signs; they confined their father in an attempt to hide his crimes. By giving him neither honor nor exit, they made him savage:[105]

---

[104] It is ironic, I think, that the members of this particular chorus seem so very tenuously linked to Thebes and yet the odes which they sing are intimately connected with the themes and even the narrative of the play. On the dramatic effectiveness of this 'detached' chorus, see discussion in Hose (1980) 143–145 and Mastronarde, *Phoenissae*, pp. 208–209. If Euripides is occasionally criticized for writing odes which appear to have little direct relevance to the matter at hand, he can hardly be said to do so in this play. For a thorough examination of the import of the odes, see Arthur (1977).

[105] On the nosological implications of this 'savageness,' see Jouanna (1988). Jouanna argues that the Hippocratic doctors may in fact have been influenced by tragic depictions of human suffering. The important notion is, he writes, 'la conception selon laquelle la maladie est une force agressive qui attaque l'individu de l'extérieur, pénètre en lui, prend possession de lui, et peut, à la manière d'une bête sauvage, se repaître de ces chairs' (344; we might note in this connection the animal imagery associated with the brothers in *Phoenissae*). Jouanna discusses the significance of the words ἀγριόω/ἀγρίος and θηριώδης in the Corpus, showing that they are particularly prominent in passages dealing with wounds and ulcers (also internal ulceration). The savageness of Oedipus' disease gives him a bestial quality, which contributes to the overall portrait of a man whose reputation for brilliance has been lost in the mire of his current dark circumstances, a man who has been removed in every possible way from the stature in the human community which he once had.

οὔτε γὰρ γέρα πατρὶ
οὔτ' ἔξοδον διδόντες ἄνδρα δυστυχῆ
ἐξηγρίωσαν· ἐκ δ' ἔπνευσ' αὐτοῖς ἀρὰς
δεινάς, νοσῶν τε καὶ πρὸς ἠτιμασμένος.   (874–877)[106]

    For giving their father neither respect
nor an opportunity to leave, they made the unfortunate old man
savage: and he breathed out his terrible curses on them,
being both sick and in addition dishonored.

Thus, the sick and dishonored Oedipus 'breathed out' curses on them, curses which have resulted not only in personal danger for his sons, but also more general danger for the city.[107] Certainly Oedipus' sons cannot be considered competent healers: they have only succeeded in exacerbating the illness by trapping it within the city.

    Tiresias offers no advice that might save the family of Oedipus. But he does reveal a mechanism by which the city itself could be saved (μηχανὴ σωτηρίας, 890) and the Argives defeated.[108] Menoeceus, Creon's son, must be sacrificed in recompense for the slaying of Ares' dragon so may years before: should blood be received for blood, then Ares will protect the city. According to Tiresias, Menoeceus' sacrifice will even act to 'cast darkness onto the eyes of the Argives' (μέλαιναν κῆρ' ἐπ' ὄμμασιν βαλών, 950). Although this action will not heal Oedipus, it will spread the suffering around. While the sacrifice of Menoeceus should no doubt be interpreted largely in the context of ritual and religious thinking, medical themes can also inform our understanding. Again, we

---

[106] These lines are part of a longer passage (869–880) that is deleted, together with 886–890, in Diggle's edition, but preserved by Mastronarde and Craik.

[107] The sickness of the land to which Tiresias refers recalls the plague which is attacking Thebes at the beginning of Sophocles' *Oedipus Tyrannus*. There, the city comes together to combat the disease that is infecting them, and they ask the clever Oedipus to help them discover the cause. When Oedipus discovers that he himself, as the incestuous patricide, is the source of the plague, he blinds himself in horror. But the fate of Oedipus at the end of the play is unclear. It is certain that he will not remain alive in Thebes, but, as I observed in Part I (p. 84), whether he suffers death or exile is left unresolved. By contrast, in *Oedipus at Colonus*, Sophocles clearly follows the tradition in which Oedipus is exiled.

[108] This notion of saving the city brings up once again the definition of that city. After all, war is not averted in the play; Thebans are killed, although to be sure, they do not lose the battle as a whole. But the sacrifice, which ostensibly pits the good of the individual family against the good of the city, seems aimed more at preserving the physicality of the city, rather than the people within. Thus, now Euripides emphasizes the geographical nature of a city, rather than its anthropological aspect. To some extent, this makes Menoeceus' sacrifice all the more poignant, in that his sacrifice saves walls rather than people.

see the use of a putatively homeopathic action that is of questionable value. Although sacrifice of like for like is demanded, Menoeceus does not match up very well with the monster in Thebes' past —he is very clearly not a dragon, even though he is descended from the dragon's teeth. Rather, he is young, innocent of marriage, pure, human—the very opposite of the dragon. Once more, we see in Euripides a complex action, one that is simultaneously homeopathic and allopathic. At 893, the action is termed a *pharmakon sôtêrias* by Tiresias, an image that Menoeceus later picks up on when he claims that his self-sacrifice will free the land from *nosos* (νόσου δὲ τήνδ' ἀπαλλάξω χθόνα, 1014).[109] While the ritual context demands a pure and untouched victim in order to atone for the violence of the past, the medical context complicates this idea—for drugs are supposed to take the evil with them as they exit the body. Menoeceus' sacrifice fails to rid the land of the Labdacids, whose presence is a source of pollution; indeed, the aim of the sacrifice is explicitly removed by Tiresias from any connection with the fate of Oedipus and his sons. Thus, this *pharmakon* fails to root out the true cause of sickness in Thebes.

In fact, despite the distinction made between the city of Thebes and the ruling house, the Thebans all pride themselves on their common ancestry, their descent from the Spartoi, the men who fought among one another until only five were left. It is impossible to differentiate entirely between the innocent and the guilty.[110] Indeed, the third stasimon reveals once again the fact that the nature of Oedipus and the nature of Thebes are very close: the chorus sings of the two-fold nature of Oedipus, who was both *kallinikos*, defeating the Sphinx, and a source of pollution, with his incestuous marriage (1043–1054). Only a few lines later, they sing of Thebes itself as *kallinika* (1059) because of Menoeceus' sacrifice; yet at the end of the verse, they note the destructive *atê* that seized the land beginning in the time of Cadmus (1065–1066). The city and the man it tried to lose when he was born are both caught in this duality of glory and destruction.

The two brothers kill one another as was ordained; Jocasta commits suicide; the Thebans manage to drive off the Argive host. The Thebans return, along with Antigone, bearing their own dead to be buried as is

---

[109] Admittedly, this line is in a section of Menoeceus' speech that is suspect and deleted by both Diggle and Mastronarde.

[110] Consider once again the implication that even Menoeceus is not entirely free from the perverse nature of the ruling house, for he was nursed by Jocasta in his infancy.

appropriate. Only now is Oedipus called forth from the house—by his daughter Antigone, who stresses once again the darkness of his existence (1534–1535). Oedipus emerges from chambers that are also dark, and learns from Antigone the unhappy fate of his wife/mother and sons. Creon interrupts their mourning and instructs Oedipus to leave the land, maintaining that his presence is a danger to it (1589–1594). After all we have been told about the threatening nature of Oedipus' diseased state, we are meant, I think, to agree that Creon's decision is the only right one, that the *apostasis* of Oedipus is essential to restoring the health of the city. Nevertheless, Oedipus resists, arguing that exile would provide the crowning touch to his miseries.[111] Creon holds firm against these arguments (1626). Unfortunately, in the next breath, he strays from the appropriate course of behavior when he refuses burial to Polyneices (1628–1630). Although we never see the outcome of this action (and it cannot be exactly the same as in Sophocles' *Antigone*, since Antigone in *Phoenissae* agrees to leave town with her father), we know that this decision will only lead to some kind of new disaster. Hence, the play ends on an ambivalent note: Antigone and Oedipus depart for the sorrows of exile; although the departure of this family has been deemed a good, Creon and the remaining Thebans nevertheless head off into an uncertain future.

Thus, the play finds no absolute remedies: perhaps the problems are simply too vast. After all, it is not merely an individual who needs treatment, but rather an entire city, an entire *genos*. Different methods are attempted: Jocasta tries gentle remedies, trying to break down the enmity of her sons with reason, with the softer methods of speech; Eteocles and Polyneices test out the methods of violence, setting up equal against equal to fight one another in battle, a mockery of their mother's belief in the peaceful force of *isotês*. Moreover, the brothers confine their sick father in an effort to conceal and to forget his crimes; but his crimes are hardly forgotten, reiterated as they are throughout the play, and this attempt to suppress him rather than to remove him results in the destruction of Eteocles and Polyneices themselves. Creon manages to do some things right, but his treatment on the one hand of

---

[111] Oedipus' speech recalls the speech of Heracles near the end of *Heracles* when he asserts that he has been unfortunate from the moment of his conception. Unlike Oedipus, however, Heracles has to be convinced to live despite his crimes, and he understands that even if he chooses to live, he must leave Thebes. In the light of this comparison, Oedipus appears selfish and unaware—hardly the image that he gives at the end of Sophocles' *Oedipus Tyrannus*.

his own son Menoeceus[112] and on the other of Oedipus' son Polyneices reveals that he is hardly reliable—he is not a consistently good healer. Only Menoeceus, whose sacrifice is mentioned just twice after it takes place, only he manages to do some good for the city—but it is surely ironic that the innocent are to die on behalf of a city apparently destined to continue its destructive ways.

d. Bacchae: *Homeopathy and repression*

If Euripides' audience had not picked up on the danger of enclosing and repressing problematic issues or individuals expressed in the *Phoenissae*, the playwright drove the point home even more clearly several years later when he composed the *Bacchae*. In this play, the danger of repression is played out once again, and, once again, on several levels. The psychological, religious, and political tensions in the play— discussed by numerous critics—are occasionally expressed in medical terms. Dionysus/the Stranger and Oedipus would seem to have little in common except for their Theban origins, yet they receive the same treatment from their misguided relatives: they are both imprisoned in attempts to rid the city of their influence. As we have seen, this course of action fails to work in *Phoenissae*: Oedipus is not forgotten; moreover, it is only as a result of his imprisonment that he directs his pain outward, cursing his sons. It is much the same case with Dionysus/the Stranger (although he has very little trouble escaping his prison): when he meets with disrespect and mistreatment, he becomes dangerous.

Pentheus maintains that the Stranger is introducing a 'new disease' (νόσον καινήν, 353–354) into the city. He attempts to eradicate this disease with violence and repression. He announces at 240–241 that he will check the activities of the Stranger by cutting off his head from his body. It is rather ironic that this surgical maneuver was consid-

---

[112] Creon's reaction to Tiresias' suggestion is surely one which elicits sympathy from a modern audience: he is horrified at the thought of sacrificing his son and encourages him to escape as quickly as possible (972). Yet Tiresias phrases the choice in terms more likely to give pause to ancient audience: he maintains that Creon can either save his family or his city (952). Many of our texts from late fifth-century Athens indicate an expectation that, at least on an ideological level, the citizen would place the good of the state before his own personal interests. Creon is inconsistent in placing the interest of his own family above those of the polis when it comes to Menoeceus, but insisting on the laws of the state when it comes to burying his nephew, Polyneices.

ered by the Greeks to be a barbarian practice,[113] while at the same
time Pentheus asserts the new religion to be barbarian/Eastern. Thus,
he will attempt to remove a barbarian religion with barbarian tactics. Horrified at the sight of his grandfather and Tiresias dressed
in Bacchic regalia, he declares that he finds nothing 'healthy' (ὑγιές,
262) in such rites. Tiresias responds with his sophistic interpretation
of Dionysus' divine existence and urges Pentheus to rethink his position on the matter. It is not those who celebrate Dionysus who are
sick, but rather Pentheus, whose judgment is disordered (ἡ δὲ δόξα
σου νοσῇ, 311: 'your opinion is sick'). Stating that he will certainly not
engage in theomachy, Tiresias ends his speech with the assertion that
Pentheus is mad. Moreover, there are no drugs by which he might
be healed—indeed, he must also be sick because of some drugs: μαί-
νῃ γὰρ ὡς ἄλγιστα, κοὔτε φαρμάκοις / ἄκη λάβοις ἂν οὔτ' ἄνευ τούτων νόσου (326–327: 'for you are mad in the most painful way possible, and neither could you find a cure through drugs nor are you
sick without them'). Tiresias no doubt says this because Pentheus is not
considered mad by nature; perhaps— although we do not know this
from the play itself—Pentheus was not always so crazy in his thinking.

What are the origins of madness? Although Tiresias seems to attribute Pentheus' madness to the impersonal force of drugs, the play
provides an alternative source of madness in Dionysus himself. The
god tells us in the prologue that he has driven the sisters of Semele
out onto the mountains, overcome with madness (32–33). Tiresias himself associates *mania* with Dionysus, specifically the *mania* of war (305).
Yet Tiresias, in his role as an advocate of rationalism, maintains that
Pentheus' madness must have some natural cause. At 283, Tiresias has
also defined Dionysus in part as a *pharmakon*—'there is no other *pharmakon* for troubles' than Dionysus (in his capacity as wine). However, at
the end of the speech, he denies that Pentheus can be cured by *pharmaka*. In these early scenes of the play, all clear notions of causality
are undermined; and we wonder about the extent to which Pentheus
is entirely responsible for his own actions, for his own 'madness.' Such
ambiguity is strengthened in Tiresias' last speech, which occurs after
Pentheus enlarges his threats against the worshippers of Dionysus. The
priest of Apollo reiterates his belief in Pentheus' madness, but indi-

---

[113] See Dodds' note *ad loc.*

cates that it has intensified: μέμηνας ἤδη· καὶ πρὶν ἐξέστης φρενῶν (359: 'you are already mad: even before you were out of your mind'). Now Pentheus is affected by that condition very much associated with Dionysus: *ekstasis*.

Pentheus' madness alters its form later in the play under the direct influence of the Stranger. When Pentheus emerges from the palace dressed as a Maenad, he is clearly deluded, making megalomaniacal claims for himself. The Stranger praises his change of mind, claiming that his thinking was not 'healthy' before, but now he thinks as he ought (947–948). Pentheus' irrational condition is defined as healthy and appropriate. Pentheus' previous state of mind, which had been defined as madness by Tiresias, stands in ironic contrast to his current condition, which the audience sees as also mad. These two forms of madness prove equally dangerous. Both the madness that Tiresias ascribes to him and the madness brought on by Dionysus are responsible for Pentheus' destruction; yet, as Tiresias points out, Dionysus only works upon what is already in a person's nature (314–318).[114] The delusions of Pentheus reveal desires repressed within his own mind and body—he had tried to lock up the Stranger, whereas it was he himself who was truly imprisoned. Dionysus acts to disclose and free the emotions within, whereas Pentheus had attempted to repress them.

The play finds no remedy for the disasters affecting its characters. Not only is Pentheus destroyed, but his family is exiled from Thebes; moreover, it seems that in his final speech Dionysus predicted the expulsion of the entire Theban folk at some point in the future.[115] Although Dionysus warns Pentheus against the wisdom of fighting evil with evil (839), he certainly confronts resistance to his cult in the most violent possible manner—indeed, Cadmus tries to rebuke him for his actions, arguing that gods should not act like men. The play thus presents a world which forces submission to dangerous and inexplicable powers from all human beings alike. It is not a consistent or predictable

---

[114] The issue of the *physis* of the family receives some attention. Three times in the play (337–340; 1227, 1291; four times if we include line 230), we are reminded of Pentheus' cousin Actaeon who suffered a fate very similar to Pentheus' fate: the former was torn apart by his own hunting dogs, the latter by his mother and aunts. And Pentheus shares his scornful attitude towards the truth of Semele's story with his mother and his aunts—skepticism is perhaps a family trait.

[115] See printed at the end of Diggle's text the fragments found in Pseudo-Gregorius, *Christus Patiens*, lines 1668–1672.

world which Euripides shows us, but it is one in which fierce repression and homeopathic-style vengeance find reward only in the world of the gods; such methods of remedy have no reasonable place in the world of mortals.

CONCLUSION

As noted in the Introduction to this study, a fragment from the comic poet Philippides seems to prescribe Euripidean tragedy as an analgesic:

> ὅταν ἀτυχεῖν σοι συμπέσῃ τι, δέσποτα,
> Εὐριπίδου μνήσθητι, καὶ ῥᾴων ἔσῃ·
> οὐκ ἔστιν ὅστις πάντ᾽ ἀνὴρ εὐδαιμονεῖ.
> εἶναι δ᾽ ὑπόλαβε καὶ σε τῶν πολλῶν ἕνα.   (fr. 18 Kassel-Austin)

> Whenever it befalls you to be unlucky in some way, master,
> remember Euripides, and you'll feel better:
> there is no man who is fortunate in all ways,
> and understand that you are one of many.

'Remember Euripides and you'll feel better,' urges the speaker; yet the comforting thought that Euripides provides is that no one is always happy.

Euripidean tragedy did not develop in isolation from Greek society and culture; presented in the context of the annual dramatic festivals, it had an integral function in the religious, social and even political institutions of fifth-century Athens.[1] Although it has not been my purpose to discuss the role of tragedy in the Athenian polis, it is important to remember, as I suggested in the Introduction, that tragedy itself was often perceived as a form of medicine (most famously, no doubt, in Aristotle's *Poetics*), an art form that was in some way to help, improve and protect the citizenry. Although Euripidean tragedy tells stories of human failure, the Athenians felt that such tragedy bestowed on them positive benefits.

The fifth century BCE has occasionally been designated 'the Greek enlightenment.' Most scholars today avoid this term and, indeed, reject the assumptions about a progression from darkness to light, from back-

---

[1] A huge scholarly literature on the function of tragedy exists; for a recent discussion, cf. Griffin (1998) with the reply of Seaford (2000). A useful and concise review of the scholarship, focusing particularly on the political aspects of tragedy, is to be found in Saïd (1998), who argues that Euripides (in contrast to Aeschylus) focuses his attention on the *oikos* and on how the demands of the *polis* undermine and even destroy the *oikos*.

wardness to civilization, from myth to reason, from belief to knowledge, that lie behind it.[2] But it is nonetheless true that some Greeks believed in this story, or, at least, believed that they were on the road of progress towards such 'enlightenment.' The writers of the treatises that were collected into the Hippocratic Corpus seem to have believed (and in some cases overtly claimed) that medicine not only benefited from that progress, but was in fact a major contributor to it.[3] Medicine, as practiced by sophisticated healers, offered to society a chance to overcome the limitations of the past, the limitations imposed on the body by the weakness of human skill in the face of disease. As the skill of medicine developed, so too would human society be able to overcome the pain and destruction that the body suffered all too easily. But, as others have argued and as I hope to have helped confirm, that story of progress is written and told in a familiar context: the tools that will bring about the new era are very often the same ones that were used in the old era. The *techne* that the healers develop uses ideas and forms of thinking that are widespread in Greek culture: cleansing and separation, change, radical or otherwise, harshness opposed to gentleness—meditations on all these topics show up repeatedly in other contemporary discourses, including, as I have argued, tragedy itself, the fifth-century genre that, with its representations of aristocratic families and archaic political structures, is perhaps the least overtly 'progressive' in its modes of communication. Tragedy absorbs and reacts to the social and intellectual currents of its own time, but it places these into the context of stories that have been running through the Greek cultural landscape for centuries.[4] Euripides, fashionably conscious of the latest trends as he seems to have been,[5] shows us the Athenian fascination with *techne* and its practitioners. The

---

[2] For an overview of the history of scholarship that sees a progression from '*mythos* to *logos*,' see Buxton's introductory remarks (Buxton [1998] 1–13).

[3] The overt message of medicine as an instrument of progress occurs in *On Ancient Medicine* 3; cf. also the claims made for the infallibility (or near infallibility) of medicine in *The Art* and *On the Sacred Disease*.

[4] This is not to say that tragedy was never subversive. Clearly, a number of factors, such the prominence and outspokenness of women in the plays and the multiple perspectives that different tragic characters afford, allow tragedy to question traditional values as well as to affirm them.

[5] Euripides was clearly a popular playwright, insofar as he was repeatedly offered a chance to put on his plays. However, whether his employment of the latest trends was 'fashionable' is perhaps debatable, given the rarity of his triumphs. On Euripides' career and reputation, see testimonia gathered in Kovacs (1994) 2–66 and discussion in the introduction to Kovacs' Loeb edition of Euripides, vol 1: 11–36.

Athenians were not famous for practicing medicine (indeed, they were well-known for employing famous healers from elsewhere, whether hiring Democedes of Croton as Herodotus tells us [3.131] or importing a cult of Asclepius from Epidaurus or, if the story is true, asking the historical Hippocrates from Cos to heal a plague);[6] but they *were* under the special protection of the technical goddess *par excellence*, Athena, and prided themselves on the superior quality of their craftsmanship, especially in the arts and in the nautical sciences.[7] Although the Athenians might also take pride in their agriculture, as they eked out a living on the meager soil of Attica,[8] their navy and their export of goods such as pottery enabled them to import a huge number of items and thus to become a center of commerce and the arts; as Pericles in Thucydides' Funeral Oration puts it, ἐπεσέρχεται δὲ διὰ μέγεθος τῆς πόλεως ἐκ πάσης γῆς τὰ πάντα (2.38.2: 'everything from every land comes in [to our city] because of the greatness of our city').[9]

'Technology' was thus an important piece of social, cultural and economic capital for the Athenians, and so it is surely not surprising to see meditations on this theme in Euripidean drama—indeed, not only meditations, but recurring themes and even structural principles, as I hope to have shown.[10] At the same time, it is not potters or ship captains who dominate the landscape in this 'technodrama,' but healers. As I have suggested, this is at least in part because of the unique nature of the healing art, which sets humans in a triangular struggle, or partnership, between healer, sufferer and disease. Unlike

---

[6] Which plague? A plague that arose sometime in 419–416, according to Jouanna (1999) 32–33. Later sources confused this plague with the plague of 430–429 described so vividly in Thucydides; for sources and discussion, see further Jouanna (1999) 31–33.

[7] In fact, the importation of skilled artists and thinkers occurs in a wide variety of fields: as Boedeker and Raaflaub (1998: 321) put it, 'apart from the dramatic poets and vase painters, relatively few leading fifth-century specialists in architecture, sculpture, monumental painting, rhetoric, historiography, science, philosophy and what is commonly called "the sophistic movement" were Athenians.' Nonetheless, as Boedeker and Raaflaub themselves argue (along with many others), the arts were essential to the functioning both of the Athenian democracy and the Athenian empire and were an integral part of the Athenian view of themselves.

[8] For the poverty of Attic soil, see Thucydides 1.2.5.

[9] On the extent of Attic trade and craftsmanship in the fifth century, see Miller (1997), with particular emphasis on exchanges with Persia.

[10] The dramatists were themselves practitioners of a *technê*, and so, perhaps, the problems and possibilities of technology were particularly close to their hearts. Moreover, like healers, their status was ambiguous, as they did earn money for their work yet also were seen to be teachers of morality and providers of wise counsel. On the ambiguous status of dramatists, see Saïd (2001).

the helmsman who must guide his inanimate ship through the wilds
of the storm, or the potter who must mold the clay and fire the oven,
or the prophet who interprets the signs given by birds or dreams, the
healer is not alone against basic matter or the wider forces of nature or
the divine: the actions and intentions of the patient, too, are involved.
The object of the healer's care is at once whole and fractured: the
disease, even when perceived as a separate entity as it so often is,
nonetheless is part of the patient's body, and thus one must go through
that body to get at the disease and induce it to come out or disperse.
The medical art is in some ways set up for failure, as Euripidean
tragedy confirms: the only healer in Euripides who successfully employs
technê to accomplish her ends is Medea, but her power is ultimately
revealed to be outside the human realm—and even so the 'cure' that
she applies hurts her as much as it hurts her target. Other healers
either mismanage their attempts completely, such as the Old Man in
Ion and the Nurse in *Hippolytus*, or they refuse to take the case, such as
Menelaus in *Orestes*, or they have patients who refuse to comply with
their directions, such as Jocasta in *Phoenissae*, whose sons will not (and,
tragically, cannot) follow her prescriptions.

Moreover, tragedy and medicine both have tales to tell. The medical
writer seeks to place the suffering patient into a *logos* of causation,
disease, and treatment; through the sophisticated systems with which
he describes the operation and the treatment of disease, he seeks to
present a closed *logos*, a completed circle of explanation and cure. The
doctor writes himself into this *logos* as the character who understands
the system and has the power to predict and even to shape the end
of the story. The tragedian, too, tells a story of suffering, in which
both the past and the present nature of that suffering are described
or portrayed with all the poetical skill the author possesses. But in
tragedy, the *logos* of suffering has no predictable end; nor is any mortal
character ever possessed of enough skill or authority to bring the story
confidently to a happy conclusion. Chance dominates the actions of
tragedy, despite the efforts of the human characters to control events.
Those characters who choose to end their stories with death find some
measure of control over their own destinies, but they can hardly be
said to have control over their own *lives*. Although there are tragedies
that do end on a positive note (where the good live on happily and
the bad unhappily), the characters are just as subject to the whims
of Tyche or the gods as their counterparts in plays with less happy
endings. Thus, while the *logos* presented in the Greek medical writers

of the fifth century is pitched as a story of empowerment, Euripidean tragedy presents more often than not a story of human weakness. While Euripidean tragedy clearly shows an awareness of, and even an engagement in, the discourse of contemporary Greek medicine, it at the same time maintains its distance, as though determined not to be seduced by the optimistic *logoi* of Hippocratic doctors. Hence (in a rebuke to the Socratic argument that if we know the good, we will choose it),[11] characters in Euripides may know the right methods but employ the wrong ones: thus, they frequently choose homeopathic methods of healing, attempt harsh remedies rather than mild ones, and fail, at least in the case of *Phoenissae*, to effect *apostasies*. Likewise, they attempt drastic changes that only create or deepen disorder, as in the case of *Heracles* or *Bacchae*. Remedies are to be found, certainly, but they are rarely the ones that the human characters expected or tried to provide.

Like the Hippocratics, Euripides is concerned with human nature and human suffering, yet he is far less optimistic than they are about the human capacity to overcome disease and suffering. The literature from late fifth-century Greece reveals to us a world in which humans were seeking new ways to explain and solve old problems; at the same time, it shows us the profound despair and pessimism with which many thinkers viewed their world. The writings of the Hippocratics and Euripides reveal to us as it were two sides of the same coin: they show us different interpretations of the search for rational explanation. It is perhaps odd that the Hippocratics, who dealt with death, disease and pain every day, were in many ways so optimistic about the human ability to find remedies for suffering—but such an attitude is fundamental to the task of science itself. And certainly it is a human characteristic to hope: indeed, even in Euripides, pessimist that he seems to be, even there, we find characters continuing to struggle against their misfortune, expressing their hope that perhaps a bond between randomness and rationalism can be forged which will reduce the pain of living.

---

[11] As formulated for us by Plato in *Protagoras* 352b–357e. Euripides' own views are not at issue here. But scholars have debated whether there was an on-going discussion between Euripides and Socrates on this principle: see Rickert (1987) 91–105 for a review of scholarly debate and Gill (1996) 226–239 for a discussion of the classical Greek poetic and philosophical approaches to the topic.

BIBLIOGRAPHY

Editions and Commentaries

Corpus Hippocraticum (arranged by date of publication)

Oeuvres complètes. vols. 1–10. ed. and trans. Émile Littré. Paris 1839–1861.

Hippocrates. vols 1–8, ed. and trans. W.H. S. Jones, E.T. Withington, W.D. Smith and P. Potter. Cambridge, Mass. 1923–1995. (= Loeb Classical Library vols. 147–150; 472–473, 477, 482)

Die hippokratische Schrift 'Über die heilige Krankheit'. ed., trans. and comm. Hermann Grensemann. Berlin 1968.

Hippokrates. Über die Umwelt. ed. and trans. Hans Diller. Berlin 1970. (= Corpus Medicorum Graecorum I 1,2)

Hippocrate. De la génération; De la nature de l'enfant; Des maladies IV; Du foetus de huit mois. ed. and trans. Robert Joly. Paris 1970.

Hippocrate. Du régime des maladies aiguës; Appendice; De l'aliment; De l'usage des liquides. ed. and trans. Robert Joly. Paris 1972.

Hippokrates. Über nachempfängnis, Geburtshilfe und Schwangerschaftsleiden. ed., trans. and comm. Cay Lienau. Berlin 1973. (= Corpus Medicorum Graecorum I 2,2)

Hippocrate. La nature de l'homme. ed., trans. and comm. Jacques Jouanna. Berlin 1975. (= Corpus Medicorum Graecorum I 1,3)

Hippocrate. Des lieux dans l'homme; Du système des glandes; Des fistules; Des hémorroïdes; De la vision; Des chairs; De la dentition. ed. and trans. Robert Joly. Paris 1978.

Hippokrates. Über die Krankheiten III. ed., trans. and comm. Paul Potter. Berlin 1980. (= Corpus Medicorum Graecorum I 2,3)

The Hippocratic Treatises 'On Generation' 'On the Nature of the Child' 'Diseases IV'. trans. and comm. Iain M. Lonie. Berlin and New York 1981.

Hippocrate. Du regime. ed., trans. and comm. Robert Joly. Berlin 1984. (= Corpus Medicorum Graecorum I 2,4)

Hippocrate. Des Vents; De l'art. ed., trans. and comm. Jacques Jouanna. Paris 1988.

Hippocrate. De l'ancienne medécine. ed., trans. and comm. Jacques Jouanna. Paris 1990.

Hippocrates: Places in Man. ed., trans. and comm. Elizabeth Craik. Oxford 1998.

'Hippocrates' *Peri Parthenión ('Diseases of Young Girls')*: Text and Translation,' Rebecca Flemming and Ann Ellis Hanson, *Early Science and Medicine* 3 (1998): 241–252.

Euripides

Euripides, Fabulae. vols. I–III. ed. James Diggle. Oxford 1981–1994.
Euripides. vols. 1–6 (Loeb Classical Library). ed. and trans. D. Kovacs. Cambridge, MA. 1994–2002.
Bacchae. ed. and comm. E.R. Dodds. Oxford 1960.
Herakles. ed. and comm. U. von Wilamowitz-Moellendorf. Berlin 1895.
Heracles. ed. and comm. G.W. Bond. Oxford 1981.
Hippolytos. ed. and comm. W.S. Barrett. Oxford 1964.
Ion. ed. and comm. A.S. Owen. Oxford 1939.
Ion. ed. and comm. K.H. Lee. Warminster, Wiltshire 1997.
Medea. ed. and comm. D.L. Page. Oxford 1939.
Medea. ed. and comm. D.J. Mastronarde. Cambridge 2002.
Orestes. ed. and comm. V. di Benedetto. Florence 1965.
Orestes. comm. W. Biehl. Berlin 1965.
Orestes. ed. and comm. C.W. Willink. Oxford 1986.
Orestes. ed. and comm. M.L. West. Warminster, Wiltshire 1987.
Phoenissae. ed. and comm. D.J. Mastronarde. Cambridge 1994.
Phoenician Women. ed. and comm. Elizabeth Craik. Warminster, Wiltshire 1988.

For other ancient works, I have generally used the editions published in the *Oxford Classical Texts* series. I have also cited from the following editions and commentaries:

Hesiod: Works and Days. ed. and comm. M.L. West. Oxford 1978.
Delectus ex iambis et elegis Graecis. ed. M.L. West. Oxford 1980.
Die Fragmente der Vorsokratiker. ed. H. Diels and W. Kranz. 6th edn. Berlin 1952.
Tragicorum Graecorum Fragmenta. ed. A. Nauck, reprint of original edition with supplements by B. Snell. Hildesheim 1964.
Tragicorum Graecorum Fragmenta. vol. 3 (Aeschylus), ed. S. Radt. Göttingen 1977.
Tragicorum Graecorum Fragmenta. vol. 4 (Sophocles), ed. S. Radt. Göttingen 1985.
Poetae Comici Graeci. vols. 4, 5, 7, ed. R. Kassel and C. Austin. Berlin 1983–1989.
Aeschylus: Prometheus Bound. ed. and comm. M. Griffith. Cambridge 1983.
Aeschylus: Eumenides. ed. and comm. A.H. Sommerstein. Cambridge 1989.
Sophocles: Oedipus Tyrannus. comm. J.C. Kamerbeek. Leiden 1967.
Herodotos: Book Two. vols. 1–3, comm. A.B. Lloyd. Leiden 1975.
Diocles of Carystus: a collection of the fragments with translation and commentary. P.J. van der Eijk. Leiden-Boston 2000–2001.
Galen: On Prognosis (= De Praecognitione). ed., trans., and comm. V. Nutton. Berlin 1979. (= Corpus Medicorum Graecorum V 8,1)
Claudi Galeni opera omnia. ed. C.G. Kühn. Leipzig 1821–1833.

Secondary Literature

Aleshire, S. (1989) *The Athenian Asklepieion: The People, their Dedicatories, and the Inventories*. Amsterdam.

Annas, J. (1993) *The Morality of Happiness*. Oxford.

Artelt, W. (1937) *Studien zur Geschichte der Begriffe 'Heilmittel' und 'Gift'*. Leipzig.

Arthur, M. (1977) 'The Curse of Civilization: the Choral Odes of the *Phoenissae*,' *Harvard Studies in Classical Philology* 81: 163–183.

Basset, L. (1995) 'L'ancien et le noveau roi (Euripide, *Heracles* 735–737, 745–746, 768–770),' *Revue de philologie, de littérature et d'histoire anciennes* 69.1: 7–14.

Belfiore, E. (1992) *Tragic Pleasures: Aristotle on Plot and Emotion*. Princeton, NJ.

di Benedetto, V. (1986) *Il medico e la malattia*. Turin.

Biggs, P. (1966) 'The disease theme in Sophocles' *Ajax*, *Philoctetes* and *Trachiniae*,' *Classical Philology* 61: 227–223.

Boedeker, D. and Raaflaub, K., eds. (1998) *Democracy, Empire and the Arts in Fifth-Century Athens*. Cambridge, MA.

Boulter, P.N. B. (1962) 'The theme of ἀγρία in Euripides' *Orestes*,' *Phoenix* 16: 102–106.

Brain, P. (1986) *Galen on Bloodletting: A study of the origins, development and validity of his opinions, with a translation of the three works*. Cambridge.

Brock, R. (2000) 'Sickness in the body politic: medical imagery in the Greek polis,' in V.M. Hope and E. Marshall, eds., *Death and Disease in the Ancient City*: 24–34. London and New York.

Burford, A. (1972) *Craftsmen in Greek and Roman Society*. Ithaca, NY.

———. (1993) *Land and Labor in the Greek World*. Baltimore, MD.

Burnett, A.P. (1971) *Catastrophe Survived*. Oxford.

Buxton, R., ed. (1998) *From Myth to Reason?* Oxford.

Cairns, D. (1993) *Aidôs: The Psychology and Ethics of Honour and Shame in Ancient Greek Literature*. Oxford.

Cairns, F. (1982) 'Cleon and Pericles: a suggestion,' *Journal of Hellenic Studies* 102: 203–204.

Chadwick, J. and Mann, W.N., trans. *The Medical Works of Hippocrates*. Oxford 1950, reprinted in G.E. R. Lloyd, ed., *Hippocratic Writings*, Harmondsworth, Middlesex 1978.

Chantraine, P. (1968; repr. 1988) *Dictionnaire étymologique de la langue grecque*. Paris.

Cohn-Haft, L. (1956) *The Public Physicians of Ancient Greece*. Northampton, MA.

Cole, S.G. (1992) '*Gunaiki ou themis*: gender difference in the Greek *leges sacrae*,' *Helios* 19: 104–222.

Cole, T. (1967) *Democritus and the Sources of Greek Anthropology*. Philological Monographs of the American Philological Association, no. 25. Cleveland, OH. [reprinted 1990 with postscript and supplementary notes. Atlanta, GA.]

Collinge, N.E. (1962) 'Medical Terms and Clinical Attitudes in the Tragedians,' *Bulletin of the Institute of Classical Studies* 9: 43–55.

Conacher, D. (1980) *Aeschylus' Prometheus Bound: A Literary Commentary*. Toronto.

Connor, W.R. (1977) 'Tyrannis Polis,' in J. D'Arms and J.W. Eadie, eds., *Ancient and Modern: Studies in Honor of Gerald F. Else*: 95–110. Ann Arbor, MI.

———. (1984) *Thucydides*. Princeton.

Cordes, P. (1994) *Iatros: das Bild des Artzes in der griechischen Literatur von Homer bis Aristoteles.* Palingenesia 39. Stuttgart.

Craik, E.M. (2001a) 'Medical Reference in Euripides,' *Bulletin of the Institute of Classical Studies* 45: 81–95.

———. (2001b) 'Plato and Medical Texts: *Symposium* 185c–193d,' *Classical Quarterly* 51.1: 109–114.

Dean-Jones, L. (1994) *Women's Bodies in Classical Greek Science.* Oxford.

———. (1995) 'Autopsia, *historia* and what women know: the authority of women in Hippocratic gynaecology,' in D. Bates, ed., *Knowledge and the Scholarly Medical Traditions*: 41–59. Cambridge.

Deichgräber, K. (1933) *Die Epidemien und das Corpus Hippocraticum.* Abhandlungen der preussischen Akademie der Wissenschaften 3. Berlin.

Demont, P. (1983) 'Notes sur le récit de la pestilence athénienne chez Thucydide et sur ses rapports avec la médecine grecque de l'époque classique,' in Lasserre and Mudry, *Formes de Pensée*, 341–353.

———. (1992) 'Observations sur le champ sémantique du changement dans la Collection hippocratique,' in J.A. Lopez Ferez, ed., *Tratados hipocraticos: estudios acerca de su contenido, forma e influencia.* Actas del VIIe Colloque international hippocratique (Madrid, 24–29 Septiembre 1990): 305–317. Madrid.

Detienne, M. and Vernant, J.-P. (1978) *Cunning Intelligence in Greek Culture and Society*, trans. Janet Lloyd. Hassocks, Sussex and Atlantic Highlands, NJ.

Diller, H. (1932) '῎Οψις ἀδήλων τὰ φαινόμενα,' *Hermes* 67: 14–42 = *Kleine Schriften zur antiken Literatur* (Munich 1971) 119–143.

———. (1934) *Wanderarzt und Aitiologie. Studien zur hippokratischen Schrift* περὶ ἀέρων ὑδάτων τόπων. Philologus Supplement 26. Leipzig.

———. (1960) 'Umwelt und Masse als dramatische Faktoren bei Euripides,' *Fondation Hardt: Entretiens sur l'antiquité classique* 6: 89–121 = *Kleine Schriften zur antiken Literatur* (Munich 1971) 335–358.

Dodds, E.R. (1951) *The Greeks and the Irrational.* Berkeley and Los Angeles.

———. (1973) *The Ancient Concept of Progress and other essays in classical antiquity.* Oxford.

Donlan, W. (1981–1982) 'Reciprocities in Homer,' *Classical World* 75: 137–175.

Dumortier, J. (1935) *Le Vocabulaire médicale d'Eschyle et les écrits hippocratique.* Paris.

Dunn, F.M. (1996) *Tragedy's End: Closure and Innovation in Euripidean Drama.* Oxford.

Edelstein, E.J. and Edelstein, L. (1945) *Asclepius: collection and interpretation of the testimonies.* Baltimore, MD. [reprinted 1998 with introduction by G.B. Ferngren]

Edelstein, L. (1931) 'Antike Diätetik,' *Die Antike* 7: 255–270 = 'The Dietetics of Antiquity,' in Edelstein, L., *Ancient Medicine* (Baltimore 1967) 303–316.

———. (1945) 'The role of Eryximachus in Plato's *Symposium*,' *Transactions of the American Philological Association* 76: 85–103 = *Ancient Medicine* 153–171.

———. (1956) 'The professional ethics of the Greek physician,' *Bulletin of the History of Medicine* 19: 391–419 = *Ancient Medicine*, 319–343.

———. (1967) *The Idea of Progress in Classical Antiquity.* Baltimore, MD.

Eijk, P.J. van der (1997) 'Towards a Rhetoric of Ancient Scientific Discourse: Some Formal Characteristics of Greek Medical and Philosophical Texts

(Hippocrates, Aristotle),' in E.J. Bakker, ed., *Grammar as Interpretation: Greek literature in its Linguistic Contexts*. Leiden.

Faraone, C.A. (1991) 'The Agonistic Context of Early Greek Binding Spells,' in Faraone and Obbink, *Magika Hiera*, 3–32.

———. and Obbink, D., eds. (1991) *Magika Hiera: Ancient Greek Magic and Religion*. Oxford.

Ferrini, F. (1978) 'Tragodia e patologia: lessico ippocratico in Euripide,' *Quaderni urbinati di cultura classica* 29: 49–62.

Foley, H. (1985) *Ritual Irony: Poetry and Sacrifice in Euripides*. Ithaca, NY.

———. (2001) *Female Acts in Greek Tragedy*. Princeton, NJ.

Foucault, M. (1985) *The Uses of Pleasure: the History of Sexuality*, trans. Robert Hurley. New York.

Garzya, A. (1997) 'Σύνεσις come malattia: Euripide e Ippocrate,' in *La parola e la scena*: 267–275. Naples.

Gill, C. (1996a) *Personality in Greek Epic, Tragedy, and Philosophy: The Self in Dialogue*. Oxford.

———. (1996b) 'Mind and Madness in Greek Tragedy,' *Apeiron* 29.3: 249–267.

———. (1998) 'Altruism or Reciprocity in Greek Philosophy?' in Gill et al., *Reciprocity in Ancient Greece*: 303–328.

Gill, C., Postlethwaite, N. and Seaford, R., eds. (1998) *Reciprocity in Ancient Greece*. Oxford.

Girard, R. (1972) *La Violence et le Sacré*. Paris.

Goff, B. (1990) *The Noose of Words: readings of desire, violence and language in Euripides' Hippolytos*. Cambridge.

Goldhill, S. (1986) *Reading Greek Tragedy*. Cambridge.

Goodman, N. (1978) *Ways of worldmaking*. Indianapolis, IN.

Gourevitch, D. (1984) *Le Triangle hippocratique dans le monde gréco-romain: le malade, sa maladie et son médecin*. Rome.

Gregory, J. (1991) *Euripides and the Instruction of the Athenians*. Ann Arbor. MI.

Griffin, J. (1998) 'The Social Function of Greek Tragedy,' *Classical Quarterly* 48.1: 39–61.

Griffith, M. (1995) 'Brilliant Dynasts: Power and Politics in the *Oresteia*,' *Classical Antiquity* 14: 62–129.

Grmek, M. (1980a) 'Le Concept d'infection dans l'Antiquité et au Moyen Age' *Rad Jugoslav. Akad. Zagreb* 384: 10–16.

———, ed. (1980b) *Hippocratica*. Actes du Colloque hippocratique de Paris. Paris.

———. (1989) *Diseases in the Ancient Greek World*. trans. M. Muellner and L. Muellner. Baltimore, MD.

Guardasole, A. (2000) *Tragedia e medicina nell' Atene del V secolo a.C.* Naples.

Hall, E. (1993) 'Political and cosmic turbulance in Euripides' *Orestes*,' in A. Sommerstein et al, eds., *Tragedy, Comedy and the Polis*: 263–285. Bari.

Hankinson, R.J. (1998) 'Magic, Religion and Science: Divine and Human in the Hippocratic Corpus,' *Apeiron* 31.1: 1–34.

Hanson, A.E. (1990) 'The Medical Writer's Woman,' in D. Halperin, J. Winkler, F. Zeitlin, eds., *Before Sexuality*: 309–337. Princeton, NJ.

———. (1991) 'Continuity and Change: Three Case Studies in Hippocratic

Gynecological Therapy and Theory,' in S.B. Pomeroy, ed., *Women's History and Ancient History*: 73–110. Chapel Hill, NC.

——. (1995) 'Uterine Amulets and Greek Uterine Medicine,' *Medicina nei Secoli—Arte e Scienza* 7: 281–299.

——. (1998) 'Talking Recipes in the Gynecological Texts of the *Hippocratic Corpus*,' in M. Wyke, ed., *Parchments of Gender*: 71–94. Oxford.

Harig, G. (1977) 'Die antike Auffassung vom Gift und der Tod des Mithridates,' *Schriftenreihe für Geschichte der Naturwissenschaft, Technik und Medizin* 14: 104–112.

——. (1980) 'Anfänge der theoretischen Pharmakologie im Corpus Hippocraticum,' in Grmek, *Hippocratica*: 223–245.

Heinimann, F. (1945) *Nomos und Physis*. Basel.

——. (1961) 'Eine vorplatonische Theorie der τέχνη,' *Museum Helveticum* 18: 105–130.

Herter, H. (1966) 'Ärtzliche Arete bei Thukydides,' *Sudhoffs Archiv* Beiheft 5: 59–69.

Hoessly, F. (2001) *Katharsis: Reinigung als Heilverfahren. Studium zum Ritual der archaischen und klassischen Zeit sowie zum Corpus Hippocraticum*. Hypomnemata 135. Göttingen.

Horden, P. (1999) 'Pain in Hippocratic Medicine,' in J. Hinnells and R. Porter, eds., *Religion, Health and Suffering*: 295–315. London and New York.

Hornblower, S. (1991) *A Commentary on Thucydides*, vol. I. Oxford.

Horstmanshoff, H.F. J. (1990) 'The Ancient Physician: Craftsman or Scientist?,' *Journal of the History of Medicine and Allied Sciences* 45: 176–197.

Hose, M. (1980) *Studien zum Chor bei Euripides*, vol. 1. Stuttgart.

Jouanna, J. (1980) 'Politique et médecine. La problematique du changement dans le *Régime des Maladies Aiguës* et chez Thucydide (livre VI),' in Grmek, *Hippocratica*: 297–319.

——. (1983) 'La sommeil médecin,' in *Théâtre et Spectacle dans l'antiquité*. Travailles du Centre du recherches sur la Proche-Orient et la Grèce antiques VII: 53–57. Leiden.

——. (1987) 'Médecine hippocratique et tragedie grecque,' *Cahiers du GITA* 3:109–131.

——. (1988) 'La maladie sauvage dans la Collection hippocratique et la tragedie grecque,' *Métis* 3: 343–360.

——. (1999) *Hippocrates*. trans. M.B. DeBevoise. Baltimore, MD.

Kallet, L. (1999) 'The Diseased Body Politic, Athenian Public Finance, and the Massacre at Mykalessos (Thucydides 7.27–29),' *American Journal of Philology* 120: 223–244.

Kerferd, G.B. (1981) *The Sophistic Movement*. Cambridge.

King, H. (1989) 'The early anodynes: pain in the ancient world' in R.D. Mann, ed., *The Management of Pain*: 56–60. Carnforth and Parkridge, NJ.

——. (1998) *Hippocrates' Woman*. London and New York.

Kirk, G.S., Raven, J.E., Schofield, M. (1983) *The Presocratic Philosophers*, 2nd. ed. Cambridge.

Kleinman, A. (1980) *Patients and healers in the context of culture: an exploration of the borderland between anthropology, medicine, and psychiatry*. Berkeley.

Knox, B. (1957) *Oedipus at Thebes*. New Haven, CT.

———. (1977) 'The *Medea* of Euripides,' *Yale Classical Studies* 25 = Knox, *Word and Action: Essays on the Ancient Theater*: 295–322. Baltimore, MD.

Konstan, D. (1999) 'What We Must Believe in Greek Tragedy,' *Ramus* 28.2: 75–88.

———. (2000) 'Altruism,' *Transactions of the American Philological Association* 130: 1–17.

Kosak, J.C. (1999) 'Therapeutic touch and Sophokles' *Philoktetes*,' *Harvard Studies in Classical Philology* 99: 94–134.

———. (2000) '*Polis Nosousa*: Greek ideas about the city and disease in the fifth century B.C.,' in V.M. Hope and E. Marshall, eds., *Death and Disease in the Ancient City*: 35–54. London and New York.

Kovacs, D. (1994) *Euripidea*. Mnemosyne Supplement 132. Leiden.

Kyriakou, P. (1998) 'Menelaus and Pelops in Euripides' *Orestes*,' *Mnemosyne* 51.3: 282–301.

Lanata, G. (1967) *Medicina magica e Religione populare in Grecia*. Rome.

Langholf, V. (1990) *Medical Theories in Hippocrates: Early Texts and the 'Epidemics'*. Berlin.

Laskaris, J. (2002) *The Art is Long: On the Sacred Disease and the Scientific Tradition*. Leiden.

Lassere, F. and Mudry, P., eds. (1983). *Formes de Pensée dans la Collection Hippocratique*. Actes du IVe Colloque international hippocratique. Geneva.

Lateiner, D. (1986) 'Early Greek medical writers and Herodotus,' *Antichthon* 20: 1–20.

Leavy, B. (1992) *To Blight with Plague: Studies in a Literary Theme*. New York.

Lefkowitz, M. (1981) *Heroines and Hysterics*. London.

Lidz, J.W. (1995) 'Medicine as Metaphor in Plato,' *The Journal of Medicine and Philosophy* 20: 527–541.

Lloyd, G.E. R. (1966) *Polarity and Analogy*. Cambridge.

———. (1979) *Magic, Reason and Experience*. Cambridge.

———. (1983) *Science, Folklore and Ideology*. Cambridge.

———. (1987) *The Revolutions of Wisdom*. Berkeley and Los Angeles.

———. (1991) *Methods and Problems in Greek Science*. Cambridge.

Longo, O. (1975) 'La polis, le mura, le navi (Tucidide, VII, 77, 7),' *Quaderni di storia* 1: 87–113.

Loraux, N. (1981) *Les Enfants d'Athèna: idées athèniennes sur la citoyenneté et la division des sexes*. Paris.

Lorenz, G. (1990) *Antike Krankenbehandlung in historisch-vergleichender Sicht: Studien zum konkret-anschaulichen Denken*. Heidelberg.

Luppe, W. (1998) 'Medizinische Unheilbarkeit von Göttern verursachter Krankheiten: zu Euripides fr. 292 N²,' in C.-F. Collatz, ed., *Dissertatiunculae criticae*:123–126. Wurzburg.

Mackie, C.J. (2001) 'The earliest Jason: what's in a name?' *Greece & Rome* ser. 2 48.1: 1–17.

Macleod, C. (1979) 'Thucydides on Faction (3.82–83),' *Proceedings of the Cambridge Philological Society* 205 ns 25: 52–68 = Macleod, *Collected Essays* (Oxford 1983) 123–139.

Maloney, G. and Frohn, W. eds. (1986) *Concordantia in Corpus Hippocraticum /
Concordance des Oeuvres Hippocratiques*. Hildesheim.

Manuli, P. (1980) 'Fisiologia e patologia del femminile negli scritti ippocratici
dell' antica ginecologica greca,' in Grmek, ed., *Hippocratica*: 393–408.

———. (1983) 'Donne mascoline, femmine sterili, vergini perpetue. La ginecolo-
gia greca tra Ippocrate e Sorano,' in S. Campese, P. Manuli and G. Sissa,
Madre Materia: Sociologia e biologia della donna greca: 147–192. Turin.

Mastronarde, D.J. (1986) 'The Optimistic Rationalist in Euripides: Theseus,
Jocasta, Teiresias,' in M. Cropp, E. Fantham and S.E. Scully, eds., *Greek
Tragedy and its Legacy*: 201–211. Calgary.

McClure, L. (1999) *Spoken like a Women: Speech and Gender in Athenian Drama*.
Princeton, NJ.

Michelini, A.N. (1987) *Euripides and the Tragic Tradition*. Madison, WI.

Miller, M.C. (1997) *Athens and Persia in the Fifth Century B.C.* Cambridge.

Müller, C.W. (1965a) *Gleiches zu Gleichem. Ein Prinzip des frühgriechischen Denkens*.
Wiesbaden.

———. (1965b) 'Die Heilung "durch das Gleiche" in den hippokratischen
Schriften *De morbo sacro* und *De locis in homine*,' *Sudhoffs Archiv* 49.3: 225–249.

———. (1993) 'Euripides, *Bellerophontes* Fr. 292 N.²,' *Rheinisches Museum* 136: 116–
121.

Nancy, C. (1983) 'ΦΑΡΜΑΚΟΝ ΣΩΤΗΡΙΑΣ: Le mécanisme du sacrifice hu-
main chez Euripide,' *Théâtre et Spectacle dans l'antiquité*. Travailles du Centre
du recherches sur la Proche-Orient et la Grèce antiques VII: 17–30. Leiden.

Nightingale, A. (1995) *Genres in Dialogue: Plato and the Construct of Philosophy*.
Cambridge.

———. (1999) 'Plato's Lawcode in Context: rule by written law in Athens and
Magnesia,' *Classical Quarterly* 49.1: 100–122.

Nussbaum, M.C. (1993) 'Poetry and the Passions: two Stoic views,' in J. Brun-
schwig and M.C. Nussbaum, eds., *Passions and Perceptions: Studies in the Hellenistic Philosophy of Mind*. Cambridge.

Nutton, V. (1983) 'The Seeds of Contagion,' *Medical History* 27. 1–34.

———. (1985) 'Murders and miracles: lay attitudes towards medicine in classical
antiquity,' in R. Porter, ed., *Patients and Practitioners*: 23–53. Cambridge;
reprinted in Nutton, *From Democedes to Harvey: studies in the history of medicine*
(London 1988), no. VIII.

———. (1992) 'Healers in the medical market-place: towards a social history
of Graeco-Roman medicine,' in A. Wear, ed., *Medicine in Society*: 15–58.
Cambridge.

———. (1995) 'The Medical Meeting Place,' in P. van der Eijk, H.F. J. Horstmanshoff, P. Schrivers, eds., *Ancient Medicine in its socio-cultural context*: 3–25.
Amsterdam.

———. (2000) 'Did the Greeks Have a Word for It?' in L.I. Conrad and
D. Wujastyk, eds., *Contagion: Perspectives from Pre-Modern Societies*: 137–162.
Aldershot, Hampshire and Burlington, VT.

Ober, J. (1989) *Mass and Elite in Democratic Athens*. Princeton, NJ.

Oberhelman, S. (1990) 'The Hippocratic Corpus and Greek Religion,' in B.
Clarke and W. Aycock, eds., The *Body and the Text*: 141–160. Lubbock, TX.

O'Brien, M.J. (1988) 'Tantalus in Euripides' *Orestes*,' *Rheinisches Museum* 131.1: 30–45.

Padel, R. (1983) 'Women: Models for Possession by Greek Daemons,' in A. Cameron and A. Kuhrt, eds., *Images of Women in Antiquity*: 3–19. Detroit.

———. (1992) *In and Out of the Mind: Greek Images of the Tragic Self*. Princeton, NJ.

———. (1995) *Whom Gods Destroy: Elements of Greek and Tragic Madness*. Princeton, NJ.

Padilla, M. (1992) 'The Gorgianic Archer: Danger of Sight in Euripides' *Herakles*,' *Classical World* 86.1: 1–12.

Parker, R. (1983) *Miasma*. Oxford.

Parry, H.P. (1969) 'Euripides' *Orestes*: the quest for salvation,' *Transactions of the American Philological Association* 100: 337–353.

Pigeaud, J. (1990) 'La maladie a-t-elle un sens?' in Potter et al., *La maladie et les maladies*: 17–28.

Plamböck, G. (1964) *Dynamis im Corpus Hippocraticum*. Abhandlungen der geistes- und sozialwissenschaftlichen Klasse (Mainz 1964), no. 2. Wiesbaden.

Porter, J.R. (1994) *Studies in Euripides'* Orestes. Leiden.

Potter, P., Maloney, G., and Desautels, J., eds. (1990) *La maladie et les maladies dans la Collection hippocratique*. Actes du VIe Colloque international hippocratique. Quebec.

Preiser, G. (1976). *Allgemeine Krankheitszeichnungen im Corpus Hippocraticum*. Berlin and New York.

Price, J. (2001) *Thucydides and Internal War*. Cambridge.

Prioreschi, P. (1992) 'Supernatural Elements in Hippocratic Medicine,' *Journal of the History of Medicine and Allied Sciences* 47: 389–404.

Rechenauer, G. (1991) *Thukydides und die hippokratische Medizin: naturwissenschaftliche Methodik als Modell für Geschichtsdeutung*. Hildesheim.

Rehm, R. (2000) 'The Play of Space: Before, Behind and Beyond in Euripides' *Heracles*,' in M. Cropp, K. Lee and D. Sansone, *Euripides and Tragic Theatre in the Late Fifth Century*. *Illinois Classical Studies* 24–25 (1999–2000): 363–375.

Rey, R. (1995) *The History of Pain*, trans. L.E. Wallace, J.A. Cadden, S.W. Cadden. Cambridge, MA.

Rickert, G. (1987) 'Akrasia and Euripides' Medea,' *Harvard Studies in Classical Philology* 91: 91–117.

Rodgers, J.A. (1969) 'Σύνεσις and the Expression of Conscience,' *Greek, Roman and Byzantine Studies* 10: 241–254.

de Romilly, J. (1976) 'Alcibiade et le mélange entre jeunes et vieux: politique et médicine,' *Wiener Studien* N.F. 10: 93–105.

Roochnik, D. (1996) *Of Art and Wisdom: Plato's Understanding of techne*. University Park, PA.

Ryffel, H. (1949) ΜΕΤΑΒΟΛΗ ΠΟΛΙΤΕΙΩΝ. Bern.

Ryzman, M. (1992) 'Oedipus, *Nosos* and *Physis* in Sophocles' *Oedipus Tyrannus*,' *L'Antiquité classique* 61: 98–110.

Saïd, S. (1985) *Sophiste et tyran, ou le problème du Prométhée enchaîné*. Paris.

———. (1993). 'Tragic Argos' in A. Sommerstein et al., eds., *Tragedy, Comedy and the Polis*: 167–189. Bari.

——. (1998) 'Tragedy and Politics,' in Boedeker and Raaflaub, eds., *Democracy, Empire and the Arts in Fifth-Century Athens*: 275–295.

——. (2001) 'Entre l'artisan et le politique: le statut social des poètes tragiques dans la démocratie athénienne,' in M. Woronoff, S. Follet, and J. Jouanna, *Dieux, héros et médecins grecs. Hommage F. Robert*: 65–96. Paris.

Salkever, S. (1994) 'Plato on Practices: the *Technai* and the Socratic Question in *Republic* 1,' in J.J. Cleary, ed., *Proceedings of the Boston Area Colloquium in Ancient Philosophy 8 (1992)*: 243–267. Lanham, MD.

Saxonhouse, A. (1992) *Fear of Diversity: the Birth of Political Science in Ancient Greek Thought*. Chicago and London.

Scarborough, J. (1983) 'Theoretical Assumptions in Hippocratic Pharmacology,' in Lasserre and Mudry, *Formes de Pensée*: 307–325.

——. (1991) 'The Pharmacology of Sacred Plants, Herbs and Roots,' in Faraone and Obbink, *Magika Hiera*: 138–174. Oxford.

Schamun, M.C. (1997) 'Significaciones de ΤΑΡΑΓΜΑ (*Perturbación*) en *Heracles* de Eurípides,' *Synthesis* 4: 99–112.

Scodel, R. (1982) 'The Second Stasimon of the *Oedipus Rex*,' *Classical Philology* 77: 214–223.

Seaford, R. (2000) 'The Social Function of Attic Tragedy: A Response to Jasper Griffin,' *Classical Quarterly* 50.1: 30–44.

Segal, C. (1992) 'Signs, Magic and Letters in Euripides' *Hippolytus*' in R. Hexter and D. Selden, eds., *Innovations of Antiquity*: 420–456. London and New York.

Simon, B. (1978) *Mind and Madness in Ancient Greece*. Ithaca, NY.

Simpson, M. (1969) 'Sophocles' *Ajax*: His madness and transformation,' *Arethusa* 2: 88–103.

Smith, B.H. (1968) *Poetic Closure: A Study of How Poems End*. Chicago.

Smith, W.D. (1966) 'Physiology in the Homeric Poems,' *Transactions of the American Philological Association* 97: 555–556.

——. (1967) 'Disease in Euripides' *Orestes*,' *Hermes* 95: 291–307.

——. (1983) 'Analytical and Catalogue Structure in the Corpus Hippocraticum,' in Lassere and Mudry, *Formes de Pensée*: 277–284.

Soter, G.M. (1993) *The Curse of Oedipus: Action and Utterance in Three Tragedians*. diss. Michigan.

Sourvinou-Inwood, C. (2003) *Tragedy and Athenian Religion*. Lanham, MD.

Staden, H. von (1990) 'Incurability and Hopelessness in the Hippocratic Corpus,' in Potter, Maloney and Desautels, *La malade et les maladies*: 75–112.

——. (1992a) 'Women and Dirt,' *Helios* 19: 7–30.

——. (1992b) 'The Mind and Skin of Heracles: Heroic Diseases,' in Danielle Gourevitch, ed., *Maladie et Maladies: histoire et conceptualisation (Mélanges en l'honneur de Mirko Grmek)*: 131–150. Geneva.

——. (1996) '"In a pure and holy way": Personal and professional conduct in the Hippocratic Oath,' *Journal of the History of Medicine and Allied Sciences* 51: 404–437.

——. (2002) 'ώς ἐπὶ τὸ πολύ: "Hippocrates" between generalization and individualization,' in A. Thivel and A. Zucker, eds., *Le normal et le pathologique dans la Collection hippocratique*. Actes du Xème colloque international hippocratique: 23–43. Nice.

Strohm, H. (1957) *Euripides: Interpretationen zur dramatischen Form*. Zetemata 15. Munich.

Taylor, J. (2000) *Framing the Past: The Roots of Greek Chronography*. diss. Michigan.

Temkin, O. (1991) *Hippocrates in a World of Pagans and Christians*. Baltimore, MD.

Thomas, R. (1993) 'Performance and Written Publication in Herodotus and the Sophistic Generation,' in W. Kullmann and J. Althoff, eds., *Vermittlung und Tradierung von Wissen in der griechischen Kultur*. ScriptaOralia 61: 225–244. Tübingen.

———. (2000) *Herodotus in Context: ethnography, science and the art of persuasion*. Cambridge.

Van Brock, N. (1961) *Recherches sur la vocabulaire médical du Grec ancien*. Paris.

Vansina, J. (1985) *Oral Tradition as History*. Madison, WI.

Vegetti, M. (1983) 'Metafora politica e immagine del corpo negli scritti Ippocratici,' in Lasserre and Mudry, *Formes de Pensée*: 459–469.

Willink, C. (1990) 'The goddess *EULABEIA* and pseudo-Euripides in Euripides' *Phoenissae*,' *Proceedings of the Cambridge Philological Society* ns 36: 182–201.

Wilson, E. (1941) 'Philoctetes: The Wound and the Bow,' in *The Wound and the Bow*: 272–295. Cambridge, MA.

Wöhrle, G. (1990) *Studien zur Theorie der antiken Gesundheitslehre*. Hermes Einzelschriften 56. Stuttgart.

Wood, E.M. (1988) *Peasant-Citizen and Slave: the foundations of Athenian democracy*. London and New York.

Worman, N. (2000) 'Infection in the Sentence: The Discourse of Disease in Sophocles' *Philoctetes*,' *Arethusa* 33.1: 1–36.

Youtie, L.C. (1996) *P. Michigan XVII: The Michigan Medical Codex (P.Mich. 758 = P.Mich. inv. 21)*. American Studies in Papyrology 35. Atlanta GA.

Zacharia, K. (2003) *Converging Truths: Euripides' Ion and the Athenian Quest for Self-Definition*. Leiden.

Zanker, G. (1994) *The Heart of Achilles: characterization and personal ethics in the Iliad*. Ann Arbor, MI.

———. (1998) 'Beyond reciprocity: The Akhilleus-Priam Scene in *Iliad* 24' in Gill et al., eds., *Reciprocity in Ancient Greece*: 73–92.

Zeitlin, F.I. (1990) 'Thebes: Theater of Self and Society,' in J. Winkler and F.I. Zeitlin, eds., *Nothing to do with Dionysos?*: 130–167. Princeton, NJ.

———. (1994) 'The artful eye: vision, ecphrasis and spectacle in Euripidean theatre,' in S. Goldhill and R. Osborne, eds., *Art and Text in Greek Culture*: 138–196. Cambridge.

INDEX NOMINUM ET RERUM

INDEX LOCORUM

I have included only passages quoted, paraphrased or directly discussed in the text.